THE
POWER
PLATE
DIET

THE
POWER
PLATE
DIET

Discover the Ultimate Anti-Inflammatory Meals to Fat-Proof Your Body and Restore Your Health

ERIN OPREA

RODALE.

New York

Published in the United States by Rodale Books, an imprint of Random House, a division of Penguin Random House LLC, New York.
rodalebooks.com

RODALE and the Plant colophon are registered trademarks of Penguin Random House LLC.

Library of Congress Cataloging-in-Publication Data
Names: Oprea, Erin, author.
Title: The power plate diet : discover the ultimate anti-inflammatory meals to fat-proof your body and restore your health / Erin Oprea.
Description: New York : Rodale, 2021. | Includes bibliographical references and index. |
Summary: "A simple, targeted diet plan that balances your plate to reduce inflammation and help you get healthy, from celebrity trainer Erin Oprea"—Provided by publisher.
Identifiers: LCCN 2020036730 | ISBN 9781984824547 (hardcover) |
ISBN 9781984824561 (paperback) | ISBN 9781984824554 (ebook)
Subjects: LCSH: Inflammation—Diet therapy. | Food habits.
Classification: LCC RB131 .O67 2021 | DDC 616/.0473—dc23
LC record available at https://lccn.loc.gov/2020036730

ISBN 978-1-9848-2454-7
Ebook ISBN 978-1-9848-2455-4

Printed in the United States of America

Photographs by Kelli Dirks
Jacket design by Anna Bauer Carr

10 9 8 7 6 5 4 3 2 1

First Edition

CONTENTS

PART 3
POWER LIVING

INTRODUCTION

Welcome to Power Plates!

If you're flipping through this book, wondering what it's all about, let me cut to the chase: This is not your typical diet and fitness book. It does not give you the same-old, same-old tips for getting in shape, such as: Cut calories? No! Kick out carbs? No! Starve yourself silly? No! Never eat your favorite foods again? No!

This plan focuses on *what you eat,* rather than on *how much you eat*—in other words, quality over quantity (as in calories). It is a "clean eating" strategy that speeds up fat-burning and makes your body *resistant* to gaining fat.

To elaborate: when the digits on your bathroom scale start creeping upward, or your clothes get really tight, you probably suspect the cause is too many doughnuts or extra scoops of ice cream. Sure, the usual bad guys—lots of junk food, too little exercise—do pack on excess flab. But there are some surprising factors that can add anywhere from a little to a whole lot of excess weight to your body. They can also throw off your hunger mechanisms and boost cravings, mess up metabolism, trigger a fat-gaining condition called insulin resistance, and cause your body to hang on to water.

These realities may both surprise you and alarm you, but trust me, Power Plates clears away these obstacles so you can drop pounds of fat without frustration, deprivation, and cravings—and keep them off over the long haul.

Since my last book, *The 4 × 4 Diet,* which was my first, I've learned more about these hidden factors and what to do about them. As a result, I developed the Power Plate Diet, a four-week plan with fat-burning menus and exercises that includes the latest research into nutrition and weight loss. On this plan, you'll learn how to incorporate a variety of clean choices into your diet, such as body chemistry–friendly foods and anti-inflammatory proteins, carbs, and fats, to get lean rapidly and without plateaus—and stay there. It gives you meal plans—my Power Plates—with easy-to-fix, delicious recipes that take away the thinking and make it easier to incorporate the right foods and the right combinations of those foods into your diet.

Power Plates work wonders, no matter whether you want better health to keep up with your kids, avoid a health condition that runs in your family, or look hot in a swimsuit or your wedding dress. No more dreaded days of reckoning in which you must wriggle into jeans or pants. No more feeling so self-conscious that you have to camouflage your body with baggy clothes. No more draggy, low-energy days.

How do I know? I'm a personal trainer who focuses on exercise *and* nutritional counseling. I'm responsible for training nearly thirty people, but not all in one day, although sometimes it feels like it. I've had countless other clients throughout my twenty-year career, too, and I've given them their own unique, individual, and focused training—each one in their own one-hour block. I've been using Power Plates with my clients for a long time, and their results are amazing. They get in great shape, look incredible, and have through-the-roof energy. Plus, the overall health effects have been nothing short of fantastic. Nearly all of my clients report that they enjoy better sleep, have glowing skin, and feel less bloated. So yes, I know it works.

Want more proof? You can see the results of Power Plates by opening up your favorite lifestyle magazine or tuning in to any red-carpet event. I've trained some of country music's most famous and fittest stars, including Kelsea Ballerini, Maren Morris, Kacey Musgraves, Jana Kramer, Carrie Underwood, Brian Kelley and Tyler Hubbard of Florida Georgia Line, Ryan Hurd, Lauren Alaina, Lee Ann Womack, Martina McBride, and Carly Pearce. Whether they're in their twenties or fifties, they're committed to a healthy lifestyle. They regularly put in the work, and it shows from head to toe, inside and out. Go ahead and admire their killer legs and toned arms, but also take note of how happy and confident they look. *That* is what Power Plates is all about.

Not all of my clients are famous faces, of course. I train people of all ages, backgrounds, and fitness levels—including my mom, who has lost ninety-six pounds! Another inspiring woman recently received her first-ever compliment on her toned legs—at the age of forty-eight! One client who wants her four-year-old daughter to grow up loving her body has used Power Plates as a way to talk about healthy eating. I have other clients who are holding off the effects of Parkinson's disease, multiple sclerosis, and other life-impairing diseases through clean eating and exercise.

I got interested in the health-giving power of nutrition long before training celebrities, however. When I was in my twenties, I enlisted in the Marines, and I served two tours in Iraq between 2003 and 2005. The day before I left for my second deployment, my friends and family gathered at my parents' house for a going-away cookout. It was during this party that tragedy struck. Suddenly and without warning, my dad fell over and died of a heart attack. He was only fifty-two!

His death was so shocking—and so unexpected because he was very active. He wasn't a bit overweight, either. I was like him, very much into the things he was into, like sports. He encouraged me to be active as a kid. I really looked up to him, and I miss him every day.

At first, I couldn't make sense of his death, but then it hit me much later, after leaving the military. Dad ate foods that were really bad for him. This made me realize that diet can be a double-edged sword—you are either feeding or fighting a disease with what you choose to eat. My dad's father died young as well, at only sixty. It can't be all genetic consequence, either, because my grandfather also ate a lot of very unhealthy foods.

After my dad passed away, I poured my time and energy into finding out everything I could about nutrition—how it can heal, energize, fight weight gain, and create longevity. His death propelled me into a whole new direction: to transform people's lives not only with exercise, but also with food. My dad is the reason I'm doing what I'm doing today—helping people live clean, lean lives through nutrition and exercise, all while making it fun.

Everything I teach my clients, and everything in this book, I've learned through a combination of hands-on experience, scientific studies and journals, and input from fellow health professionals. All of this has taught me that a lot of what's going on with your weight isn't always your fault. That's not to say you have no power to control it. You have enormous power! That's why I named this plan "Power Plates"; it's made up of power foods that make up perfect, fat-burning meals.

FAT-PROOF YOUR BODY. A big reason why you've probably struggled with your weight has to do with the function of your fat cells. If they're inflamed or irritated by the wrong foods, they simply cannot release fat. Fat gets trapped inside cells and is virtually impossible to budge. The solution is to avoid these offending foods and instead select clean foods that will help your fat cells shrink so you get lean and fit. Choosing the right foods can help you drop pounds—up to three to five pounds a week—which is what I've observed with my clients, especially when coupled with exercise. The essence of proper food selection is what I tell my clients all the time: Eat responsibly and think before you eat.

ENJOY BALANCED EATING, WITHOUT DEPRIVATION. When people find out I'm a personal trainer and a diet book author, they always ask, "So what do you think about the [you fill in the blank] diet?" And so the conversation goes . . .

Let me say that it's not my job to judge. In my heart of hearts, I'm okay if you're a vegan, a keto fan, or a paleo convert. What I'm not okay with are diets that are unsustainable and unbalanced, or plans that eliminate whole food groups, or don't consider your personal body chemistry. On those fads, you feel great when you drop a size or two, then beat yourself up when you gain five or ten or more pounds after going back to old, bad eating habits. Or you try to deprive yourself skinny, and your body breaks down muscle for fuel. You are literally eating yourself alive. Or you're unknowingly feeding yourself with inflammatory, reactive foods that keep you from losing weight. These issues cause untold physical and emotional problems.

I want you to enjoy your life! I want you to eat a balanced diet from all the food groups, with your favorite foods included at times. One of my mottoes is "everything in moderation." So within reason, I allow indulgences here and there. I love doughnuts, for example, but I don't have them around too often—and only when I walk to get them (which could be a six-mile walk). How much do I love doughnuts? My husband, Sean, and I almost bought a building in Nashville to start a doughnut shop—until the March 2020 tornado destroyed it.

I'm serious when I say that for every deprivation diet there is an equal and opposite splurge. Science backs me up on this: University of Toronto researchers have found that dieters who are deprived of their favorite foods eventually respond by bingeing on those foods and regaining weight, with interest.

Deprivation doesn't work. People want what they can't have, so when you eliminate a favorite food from your diet, you only crave it more. Life isn't just one big diet!

EXPERIENCE BOUNDLESS ENERGY. I get it that you're mainly interested in attaining your ideal weight. But you can't get there if you're energy-challenged and too tired to put in the work. I know I couldn't be where I am today without energy. I'm up and ready to rock at 3:30 every morning with my belly growling, ready for my breakfast of oatmeal, egg whites, and berries. By 4:30 a.m., I'm heading out the door to meet my first client of the day. I work with clients in their homes, usually about ten people throughout the day, and when I'm driving in between, I eat, run my business, and give interviews on the phone (and sometimes I get to make a pit stop!).

I get home around four or five o'clock, and eat a clean dinner with food that my husband and I prepped on Sunday. Some nights, I have meetings or interviews, or a photo shoot. Or I'll hit the gym and work on my Instagram posts. There are a few evenings when I attend red-carpet events or concerts with my clients. Life is full!

I usually go to bed at about 10, then hit it all over again! (I know that's not enough sleep—that's my downfall.) But my point is: This is what an energized life looks like. With the right foods, hydration, and exercise, you can go from dragging to doing! There's no way I could keep up this schedule without properly fueling my body.

MAKE EXERCISE FUN. Power Plates includes some fun exercises to help you create body-firming muscle and obtain results even faster. Yes, you read that right: *fun exercises*. My approach is making every workout enjoyable. I do this through special games you can play as part of your workout, performing variations of simple exercises, having the freedom to work out in the comfort of your home, and blasting great music at the highest level (music is the key to any successful workout, in my opinion). I love making fitness fun. The routines here deliver that fun.

There's more to it, though. Exercise has more of an anti-inflammatory effect than anyone ever knew. Moving around sends out a blast of anti-inflammatory proteins from your cells to the rest of your body.

TRANSFORM YOUR LIFE. When you alter your body shape for the better and are feeling energized, something happens to the way you feel about yourself, your relationships, and your whole way of being in the world. Seriously, those lost pounds are replaced with new, powerful feelings of self-control, better health and fitness, smaller-sized clothing, lots of compliments, hope, excitement, and an overall burst of self-worthiness. I've not yet met anyone who successfully made over their body without finding that their lives changed in ways—incredible ways—that they never imagined. I can't wait for this to happen to you!

It's so easy to sit around and say, "I want to be able to do this. I want to be able to look like that. I want to feel good." The hardest part is making the decision to actually make the change. I'm going to show you that when you feel amazing, you'll never want to go back to your old habits. You'll get to a point where every night you look forward to waking up the next morning rather than being excited at the prospect of sleeping in. You'll feel so good on the inside and out that you won't want to ruin that feeling. You'll want to keep going. And you will keep going.

Everything I've ever done has been leading, pushing, and guiding others to reach their goals. Now that we've met on these pages, I want to see you succeed and really turn your life around. Embrace the Marine Corps motto: *Semper Fidelis* ("Always Faithful"). Taken to a personal level, it means always be faithful to yourself—your goals, dreams, health, and the life you truly want. Start living that way today. It will be the first day of a new, fit life leading to a healthier future. You have absolutely nothing to lose—and so much *power* to gain.

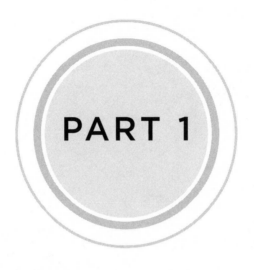

PART 1

LOSE WEIGHT NATURALLY

1

BE FAT-PROOF!

Let me sum up what Power Plates will do for you: *fat-proof your body.*

A fat-proofed body is one that easily burns fat, including belly fat, and is resistant to gaining or regaining fat pounds. You might say that a fat-proofed body operates like that of your naturally fit friends. We all have them—people who share a combination of traits such as a fast metabolism, a modest appetite, great blood sugar control, and a smaller tummy size. You are about to join their ranks.

How is this possible? Basically, Power Plates reprogram your fat cells so that you burn fat, day in and day out. You keep losing inches and pounds right down to your ideal shape and weight, without the plateaus you've experienced on other diets. This happens because you'll be healing your fat cells so that they burn off stored fat the way they're supposed to. The more you fat-proof your body, the more easily excess pounds will melt off. You'll feel and look so much lighter and have an absurd amount of energy.

The Secret Life of Fat Cells

When you see your naked reflection in the mirror, you're looking at a mix of cells. Many of them are fat cells, sandwiched between skin and muscle cells. We have approximately seventy-five billion fat cells. When healthy and operating like they should, they are about the size of a period at the end of a sentence.

From birth to your early twenties, the number of fat cells on your body increases. But when you reach your mid-twenties, the number of fat cells remains constant. Fat cells do die off, but the body quickly replaces them.

Under a microscope, a fat cell resembles a fried egg on top of a beach ball of fat. Most of the cell's bulk is triglycerides, a fat that's chemically similar to diesel fuel. The remaining non-fat part of the cell includes organelles involved in metabolism—the body's food-to-fuel process.

Fat cells used to be thought of as an inactive, jiggly mass that took up space and made our waistline expand. But now we know that fat tissue is far more active and has important jobs in the body. For one thing, fat is the largest endocrine (hormone-producing) organ in the body. It sends out messages via hormones to the brain and other parts of the body that have to do with hunger and appetite. For example, healthy fat triggers weight-control hormones, such as leptin, to tell your brain that you've had enough food.

Normal fat cells are used by the body to store energy—in some cases for several months at a time. The energy you'll use to do my exercise routine today may be coming from that cheeseburger you ate two months ago. Every excess calorie that your body does not burn up is kept in the fat cells—even the calories from celery or carrots.

It's not the number of fat cells that dictates your weight; it's their size, which can fluctuate depending on how much fat they're storing. When you lose weight, the size of your fat cells shrinks. There is no guarantee that they will stay small, however, especially if you revert to a bad diet or stop working out.

When you gain weight or eat unhealthy food, fat cells inflate. This restricts normal blood flow to the cells and stops them from functioning normally. They pack away fat at an excessively high rate and release fat at a terribly slow rate. What's more, swollen fat cells churn out abnormal amounts of various hormones. At abnormal levels, these hormones worsen inflammation—which is a big cause of more fat gain—and slow down metabolism. More fat is then crowded into fat cells, leading to bloated, unhealthy toxic cells that continue to store fat and hold on to it for dear life.

The larger your fat cells, the harder it can be to drop weight. This gets to be a vicious cycle, especially if you don't exercise much and eat too much of the wrong foods. We're going to break that cycle now—and stop producing bigger fat cells that make future weight-loss efforts so tough.

Power Plates Help Fat Cells Properly Release Fat

Let's talk about how Power Plates work. Primarily, they "cool" inflammation, a process I'll talk about in detail in the next chapter. But for a summary, inflammation is the body's natural response to protect itself against harm. Normally, it works in the short term to heal injuries and illnesses, then shuts off. But if it doesn't shut off, inflammation causes many serious diseases—even obesity. If someone eats a lot of processed food, junk food, sugar, or foods to which they're intolerant or allergic, this food inflames their fat cells and those cells act like they're infected. As a consequence, they will not release fat. They will stubbornly hoard it, so it can't be burned. Fat cells then inflate and get bigger. This is the reason people pack on pounds—enlarged fat cells. Inflammation is thus a huge threat to fat cells and prevents us from losing body fat. So, unless this situation is resolved with proper diet and exercise, someone can become overweight or obese.

Excess body fat, especially around your tummy, is an *additional* risk factor for inflammation. This turns into another vicious cycle. But by following Power Plates, you protect your fat cells from inflammation so that they perform their job of releasing fat so that it can be burned.

The Food Sensitivity Connection

Here's a biggie when it comes to weight control: food sensitivities. An important part of cooling inflammation is to identify your food sensitivities and cut back on foods that make you feel sick. Nearly 20 percent of us have some type of food sensitivity. This causes a reaction in the body that can trigger weight gain (especially around the middle), cravings, and bloating. Eating reactive foods regularly makes it harder to burn off fat and get lean.

I've observed this phenomenon in many of my clients—even in myself. A few years ago, I'd sauté lots of veggies, including onions, for dinner. Within thirty minutes, my stomach would bloat so much that my sons thought I was pregnant. There would be wicked gas (it's a good thing my husband and I could laugh that off). I'd get headaches, too, along with swollen finger joints. I felt like I had the flu.

I was miserable, so I took a food sensitivity test. First of all, it turned out that my body can't tolerate yeast. It affected me worse than any other food. That meant no more pizza. I was pretty miserable over that until I discovered yeast-free cauliflower-crust pizza. Second, my other sensitivities were to potatoes and onions (which were triggering my bloat and discomfort). Goodbye potatoes and onions—and gas. Hello to a happier husband.

Once I cut out these reactive foods, especially yeast, my symptoms vanished. If you've experienced something similar, know that I'm here for you. There's real evidence that addressing this key cause of weight gain can help you shed pounds. This plan can be a powerful tool to help you learn which dietary changes can produce dramatic effects in weight loss and overall health.

Power Plates Provide Fat-Burning Meal Combos

In addition to cooling inflammation and controlling reactive foods, Power Plates are made up of mixed meals of proteins, carbohydrates, veggies, and fat, in the right combinations to help you lose weight, control cravings, and fat-proof your body.

Our bodies evolved on a diet of mixed meals of protein, carbohydrates, and fat. Therefore—because many foods contain a combination of these macronutrients—your digestive tract is always prepared to digest a mixed meal. There are several advantages of eating like this. Mixed meals:

BOOST THE "THERMIC EFFECT OF FOOD" (TEF). This is the rate at which your body burns calories after you eat. It accounts for at least 10 percent of your daily energy expenditure.

Not all macronutrients are created equally when it comes to TEF. Some types of food help your body burn more energy than others. Protein and natural, high-fiber carbohydrates have a TEF of 25 percent (good), while fats have a TEF of 5 percent (bad). Eating junk food like candy bars or toaster pastries will give you a TEF of only 3 percent (horrible). Not very helpful, I think you'll agree! The Power Plates mixed meals help boost your TEF.

SUPPORT FAT LOSS. Power Plates feature a combination of protein, carbs, vegetables, and fat, so the nutrients in them break down slowly. This reduces the surge in blood sugar, creates energy at a steady rate, and stabilizes weight-control hormones after meals—all factors that put your body in a fat-burning mode throughout the day.

By contrast, if your blood sugar zooms up—the result of improper food combinations (like too many carbs and sugary foods)—your body responds by making excess insulin. Yes, insulin is related to diabetes, but we all produce this important hormone. It allows the body to use sugar (glucose) from carbohydrates in the food that we eat for energy or to store glucose for future use. Insulin helps keep our blood sugar level from getting too high (hyperglycemia) or too low (hypoglycemia). Too much insulin accelerates the conversion of excess calories into body fat. Power Plates help regulate blood sugar and blunt insulin in your body safely and naturally so that you can lose weight while eating a full range of foods.

In fact, a study carried by the *Journal of the American Medical Association* (JAMA) found that dieters who wanted to maintain their weight loss burned significantly more fat and kept the weight off longer using proper meal combos of protein, carbohydrates, vegetables, and a little fat.

MANAGE HUNGER. I used to wonder why I'd feel full after a breakfast of oatmeal and scrambled eggs, but I could eat three doughnuts and still want more. Well, it has to do with something called "satiety." It's a buzzword used in nutritional circles. It means a state of feeling full.

Protein and high-fiber carbs and veggies have a very high satiety rating. So when you eat them together in a mixed meal, you'll feel full longer. Power Plates are designed with this in mind. They help curb your hunger and prevent food cravings.

SUPPORT YOUR HEALTH. There are health benefits of mixed meals, too. Certain nutrients, such as fat-soluble vitamins (vitamins A,

D, E, and K) and carotenoids, require some fat in order to be absorbed by the body. Carotenoids are disease-fighting plant chemicals found in red, orange, and dark green veggies like carrots, tomatoes, red bell peppers, spinach, and broccoli. So when you fix a salad of these veggies and drizzle it with olive oil, the combination helps your body absorb the nutrients in them so much better. Another example is mixing foods high in vitamin C (such as lemons or bell peppers) with plant-based sources of iron like spinach or beans. The vitamin C helps your body absorb the iron. So squirting lemon juice on your greens is a super-healthy idea.

Power Plates Versus the Keto Diet

Let's take a little detour here. When I mention "fat-burning," what often comes to mind is the trendy keto diet, in which the body uses fat as fuel. The Power Plate diet rids your body of unsightly fat, too, but goes about it in an entirely different way than keto does, plus has different nutritional principles. The differences:

THE METABOLICS. The main factor with the keto diet is that it pushes people to eat fewer carbs and ramp up their fat intake. The keto diet gets the body into "ketosis." This is the condition in which the body burns fat for fuel instead of carbohydrates. In order to do that, most keto diets recommend that you stick to about 40 grams of carbs or less per day, which means that there's not much room for fruits and many vegetables.

I agree that limiting carbs does have a fat-burning effect. But you don't have to cut them out entirely, or go all day without carbs. You can achieve the same fat-burning benefit on the Power Plate Diet with my Modified Carb Fast. I'll explain this later, but it involves not eating any high-carb foods past 3 or 4 p.m. Essentially, you go from the afternoon until the next day's breakfast without starchy carb foods—roughly fifteen to sixteen hours. During this time (most of which you're asleep), your body gets an additional opportunity to burn more fat—without following a highly restrictive keto diet!

THE NUTRIENT MIX. The two styles of eating are built on a foundation of different food groups. The ketogenic diet is based on a pattern of high-fat foods, moderate protein choices, and a very low quota of carbs. It tends to be quite limited, with a long list of foods you can't eat.

Power Plates, on the other hand, emphasize whole grains, legumes, fruits, and other fiber-rich carbohydrate foods. These food groups provide a lot of anti-inflammatory power to keep your fat cells doing their job—releasing fat and shrinking in the process. The keto diet does not emphasize these nutrient-rich food groups.

Very few foods are off-limits on the Power Plate Diet. But with keto, there are certain foods that you aren't permitted to eat or don't have room to eat because your carb grams are so restricted. Power Plates let you work in many more foods. This keeps you on the plan, with fewer cravings and yearnings for certain foods, whereas restrictive diets are hard to stick to and make you want to overindulge in foods you miss.

DIETARY FAT ISSUES. Both diets allow foods with fat, but not really the same types of fats. People on the keto diet may find themselves eating fatty foods like cheese, bacon, and butter. I don't have a problem with any of these foods. They're tasty in moderation. I love a little bacon crumbled on a salad with a sprinkling of cheese, occasionally.

What's risky is the type and amount of fat permitted on a keto diet. It tends to be high in saturated fat, which is highly inflammatory and thus can inflame fat cells, hindering their ability to release fat. The keto diet also emphasizes fats so much that it can be challenging to get adequate amounts of other big nutrients, such as healthy carbs and lean proteins. Any diet high in saturated fat is going to cause cholesterol problems, too. I've had clients who followed the keto diet and now have high cholesterol as a result. You can't gobble up large amounts of meat, cheese, and fat without consequences.

The Power Plate Diet takes a more measured approach to fat choices. It focuses on anti-inflammatory, healthier fats like avocados, olive oil, and omega-3 fats—all in moderation.

NO COUNTING. I like things simple! The keto diet requires you to keep track of your macronutrients. To stay in ketosis, you have to tally up grams of carbs, grams of protein, grams of fat, and be a human calculator when it comes to eating.

Power Plates take much less planning than the keto diet, and the emphasis is really on foods over numbers. You simply design your plate with combinations of macronutrients. No counting! While you do have to stay focused on your portion sizes, it's easy with Power Plates.

THE PERMANENCE OF WEIGHT LOSS. Both the keto diet and Power Plates promote weight loss, but keeping it off is a different story. When you stop keto dieting and go back to eating carbs, you can regain your lost weight with interest, because you have altered your body's metabolism.

The better dietary solution is a balanced meal plan like the Power Plate Diet that includes a range of healthy foods, including carbs, put together in the right combinations.

Specific Nutrients That Fat-Proof Your Body

A number of specific nutrients are required to keep a fat cell happy and functional—and your body in fat-proofing mode. Here's an overview of how the nutrition in Power Plates reboots your fat cells and metabolism so that your body burns fat properly.

1. POWER PLATES ARE RICH IN POWER PROTEINS.

Very simply, a "protein" is generally anything that once walked, flew, or swam (although there are many plant-based proteins, also). I call them power proteins because they help burn fat and create body-firming muscle.

Two of my favorite proteins are poultry and fish. We all know they're healthy but here's why: They're high in an amino acid called taurine. It's really good at squelching inflammation in fat tissue and keeping fat cells healthy. It boosts helpful cellular substances that empower fat cells to release fat and stimulate weight loss.

Incidentally, research has found that obese people have low levels of taurine in their bodies. We need ample taurine and other amino acids from protein to make our fat cells happy.

Protein in general triggers fat-burning, particularly around the belly. Several studies have substantiated this, although it's not clear why protein is so good at trimming off unsexy belly fat. Scientists think it has to do with protein's ability to rev up metabolic rate. Belly fat burns off pretty quickly in response to a higher metabolism. Compared with other fat storage sites on the body, the abdominal region gives up fat easily.

Protein also keeps you full and tames food cravings. Research published in the journal *Obesity* in 2011 proved that a higher protein intake promotes satiety (fullness), plus preserves fat-burning lean muscle as you lose weight, which is critical for achieving the body you want.

2. POWER PLATES EMPHASIZE POWER OMEGA-3 FATS.

Found mostly in fish and other seafood, these fats have several fat-burning benefits. First, they work within the fat cell to cool the inflammation that irritates those cells and makes them cling to fat.

Second, omega-3s boost an enzyme called lipase. Remember the old video game Pac-Man? Lipase is like Pac-Man. It runs around and chomps away at fat in cells, snipping it into little pieces called fatty acids. Those fatty acids are then released in the bloodstream, which carries them to muscle cells where they are burned for energy. Greater lipase activity is a marker of good fat cell health, while low lipase activity sets the stage for obesity.

Third, omega-3s guard fat cells from the damage caused by junk food, which makes fat cells enlarge and shifts the body into a fat-gaining mode.

It's preferable to get your omega-3s from whole foods such as fish because they are better absorbed by the body. And chia seeds, flax-seeds, and walnuts are good plant sources of these nutrients. So you definitely want to populate your diet with these amazing fat-burning and inflammation-busting fats!

3. POWER PLATES PERMIT POWER CARBS.

A carb, generally, is anything that once grew in the ground or is made from something that once grew in the ground, such as whole-wheat pasta. Carbs can and should be your friends (I mean, let's get a big round of applause!). They are fantastic! In fact, you need carbs to help shed fat, particularly belly fat. But not just any carbs—natural, clean carbohydrates. I call them power carbs. They are rich in fiber and therefore release energy into the bloodstream slowly. This prevents spikes in insulin and blood sugar that, when stored and stockpiled, pack inches around your waistline.

Power carbs that I adore include oatmeal, brown rice, beans and legumes, and sweet potatoes. Some—like quinoa—are gluten-free, and thus help prevent irritating tummy bloat. These are examples of quality carbs, which are super-essential for healthy fat cells.

With Power Plates, you'll learn to time your carbs, too, for best results. I don't recommend starchy carbs like pasta, potatoes, or bread on your dinner plate, for instance. There's just no reason to eat those types of carbs in the evening. Carbs are energy foods, and you don't need them while you're sleeping. Cutting them out in the late afternoon and at night, using my Modified Carb Fast, accelerates fat-burning and creates drastically attractive results in your physique.

Have all those healthy carbs—just earlier in the day. Don't eliminate them!

4. POWER PLATES ARE FULL OF POWER PRODUCE.

Some of the most anti-inflammatory foods you can eat are plant-based—vegetables, fruits, nuts, seeds, herbs, and spices. These are a rich payload of vitamins, antioxidants, and disease-fighting natural chemicals, all with anti-inflammatory properties that protect our cells, including fat cells. Plus, they give your meals so much flavor! Healthy food shouldn't be boring. EVER.

I haven't met an herb or a spice that I don't like. They are concentrated sources of anti-inflammatory components. In fact, roughly two tablespoons of most spices contain as many health-promoting antioxidants as ten servings of fruits and vegetables. You can also find low- or no-sodium spices that add a lot of flavor to foods and help you keep your salt intake in check.

After you put together your Power Plates, you'll see that they are very colorful. The more color on your plate—red, dark green, orange, purple—the more you'll help your body's natural defense system stop inflammation.

5. POWER PLATES FOCUS ON NUTRIENTS OVER CALORIES.

It's certainly true that you can ignore your hunger pangs, white-knuckle it out on a starvation-type diet, and drop pounds. But in terms of things we can tolerate without going crazy, it makes a lot more sense to eat delicious, filling foods that will stimulate your fat cells to release more fat. That's what I do—I eat a lot of super-healthy foods that supply my body with loads of nutrients.

This is where *diet quality* enters the picture. Diet quality describes clean, nutrient-rich meals—foods that have the most nutrients and anti-inflammatory substances for the least calories. For example, let's compare a baked potato with a cupcake. Both have about 170 calories, but the nutrient counts are vastly different. The baked potato has four times as much fiber and much less sodium. It provides 22 milligrams of vitamin C (a great inflammation fighter); the cupcake contains very little fiber and vitamin C and has six times more empty-calorie sugar. We'd have to eat a lot of cupcakes (and calories) to match the nutritional value of a baked potato. But be careful to not downgrade the nutritional wealth of a baked potato by loading it up with sour cream, cheese, and bacon. I can see your mind working those angles!

The quality of the calories you eat has a greater impact on your health than the quantity. Keep my favorite motto in mind: *Calories are not created equal.* One hundred calories of oatmeal versus one hundred calories of sugary ice cream don't compare, nutrient-wise. So rather than obsess over calories, it's better to focus on the nutrients in your food—diet quality—to prep your fat cells for easier weight loss and better metabolic health. When you shoot for diet quality with Power Plates, you have lots and lots of foods to choose from. Your meals will never be bland or boring.

Plating It Up!

When it comes to getting in shape, three (or more) foods are better than one. That's because each type of food has different nutrients that work together. As a team, they fend off cravings, help you stay full longer, and burn fat better than they would solo. So when you combine power proteins, power carbs, power veggies, and power fats on your plate, you've just created a meal geared for steady fat loss!

Summing up, with anti-inflammatory foods and the right meal combos, you'll burn up fat that is already stored on various parts of your body and produce rapid results to give you the motivation to continue losing weight all the way down to your goal. The Power Plate Diet is extremely effective for getting lean quickly because you coax your body into using fat as its primary fuel source—and the result is more rapid weight loss.

Power Plates thus transform your fat cells into a more metabolically healthy, fat-loss state. Essentially, this plan gets your fat cells to act like those of a fit and healthy person. This makes weight loss and optimal health easier—and is the reason why Power Plates work.

HOW EXERCISE FAT-PROOFS YOUR BODY

While Power Plates mount a pretty powerful resistance against fat gain, so does exercise, especially weight training. I'm not necessarily talking about weights, barbells, or machines, although these are awesome and I use them with my clients all the time.

Know this: Your body is also weight, and you can use it to create attractive muscles. And muscle is key to metabolism. The more muscle you have, the faster your metabolic rate is—that is, the rate at which your body burns calories at rest, even while you're sitting on your couch, watching Netflix. It's a win-win.

Developing lean muscle is really important because after age thirty you may lose half a pound of muscle each year, unless you exercise. At the same time, you may gain about one and a half pounds of body fat a year—much of it as belly fat. So if you lose pounds of muscle over the years, calories don't get burned the way they should, and fat is created and deposited. You've got to work your muscles to fat-proof your body.

Of course, there are several ways to do this. In addition to body weight training, I like Tabata workouts, which you'll do on this plan. More on this later, but they combine both strength and cardio work into one simple—and shorter—routine that I turn into a series of fun games.

You can add in other cardio activity, too. It is essential to weight control (including burning belly fat) and heart health. You can walk 10,000 daily steps easily and naturally. Or do any type of cardio you enjoy. For me, a jump rope is my best friend. Jumping rope is serious business—and it gets body-shaping results faster than a long, hard run. It doesn't cost much, either. Find what makes you happy and challenges you.

Worth emphasizing, too, is that oodles of studies show that exercise—and its chief effect, fitness—lower markers of inflammation. The way exercise does this is by reducing body fat, lowering blood pressure, improving sleep, and enhancing glucose metabolism, to name just a few perks.

Our bodies are made to move. If we don't move them, they break down. The same thing happens with our cars. If you don't move a car for a long time, it doesn't want to start. The more you move, the better you'll feel.

2

THE WEIGHT-INFLAMMATION CONNECTION

When it comes to fat-proofing your body, we need to dig into a big obstacle standing between you and a completely fit and healthy existence: inflammation. Affecting nearly 60 percent of the U.S. population, it is directly related to the food you eat and the quality of your diet.

Now's a good time for a confession. A couple of years ago, I wouldn't have been able to write a paragraph about inflammation, let alone an entire chapter of a book. I paid as much attention to inflammation as I did to *The Bachelor*—which is to say none at all. But as time went by, I started hearing about it from my clients. I realized it was something we don't want floating around in our bodies. When I learned that inflammation is a major hidden cause of weight gain, I was shocked!

Over the past couple of decades, researchers have been ramping up studies and discovering the link between inflammation and many, if not most, common diseases. And recent findings tie inflammation closely to overweight and obesity. In fact, both conditions are character-ized by inflamed fat cells. Before we unpack that connection, let's start with Inflammation 101.

Inflammation: The Good and the Bad

Inflammation is one of your body's most powerful feats. In simple terms, it is a natural defense mechanism that leaps into action whenever your body perceives a threat, like an injury or an infection. When everything is working properly, inflammation puts you on the fast track to recov-ery. This process is absolutely crucial for your body to heal properly.

Sounds great, right? Unfortunately, inflammation can be two-faced. Not all inflammation is healthy, helpful, or a sign of healing. Just like fats and cholesterol, there are "good" and "bad" kinds of inflammation. Both involve your immune system, which serves as your body's security detail against all kinds of threats, but they have drastically different ef-fects on your body.

Acute Inflammation

The "good" kind of inflammation is acute inflammation. Whenever your body detects something that is trying to harm it—an injury, infec-tion, virus, illness, toxin, or stress—your immune system dispatches an army of specialized white blood cells to fix the problem.

Let's say you stub a toe, get a bee sting, twist an ankle, get scratched by an excited dog, or experience a paper cut by opening a doughnut box too fast. Or maybe you come down with a cold or the flu. In cases like these, your immune system immediately sends those blood cells on a mission to surround, protect, and heal the affected area. With a cold or the flu, white blood cells are instructed to prevent the viruses and any potential bacteria from spreading.

You know when you're experiencing acute inflammation because its symptoms are easy to see and feel. As your blood cells rush to the site of the injury or illness, they produce any combination of redness, pain, swelling, heat, and loss of function. These symptoms vary depending on the type of injury or infection and where it occurs.

In short, acute inflammation is how we heal. Without it, your body would be largely defenseless against even tiny scrapes and random dust particles; wounds and diseases would fester, and infections could become deadly. Because acute inflammation is a sign that your immune system is in fight mode, working to fend off threats to your body, usually you can just wait it out until you've healed yourself within a matter of hours or days—this is your body using its power for good. Acute inflammation is like a flash fire that ignites instantaneously, remains contained, and extinguishes quickly, all in order to protect your body.

Chronic Inflammation

Whereas acute inflammation is the good kind of inflammation, chronic inflammation is the bad, harmful kind. It's also known as "non-resolving inflammation" and "persistent, low-grade inflammation" because it produces a constant hum of inflammatory responses throughout the body—and those can lead to long-lasting conditions like heart disease, diabetes, and even cancer. Chronic inflammation is proof that there can be too much of a good thing. And chronic inflammation is what we're combating with Power Plates.

MAJOR DISEASES LINKED TO CHRONIC INFLAMMATION

ALLERGIES: These are the sixth leading cause of chronic diseases in the United States and affect more than fifty million Americans each year.

ARTHRITIS AND JOINT DISEASES: These conditions affect nearly 43 million people in the United States or almost 20 percent of the population.

CANCER: The American Cancer Society reports that the rate of new cancer cases diagnosed each year is around 1.8 million, with nearly 607,000 deaths annually.

CARDIOVASCULAR DISEASES: These account for one out of every three deaths or approximately 800,000 deaths a year in the United States. My dad was one of these tragic statistics—which is why health and nutrition matter so much to me.

CHRONIC OBSTRUCTIVE PULMONARY DISEASE (COPD): This is a lung disease—and the third most common cause of death in the United States.

DIABETES: This disease is the seventh leading cause of death in the United States.

OBESITY: More than two in three adults are overweight or obese. Nearly 14 percent of children and teens are considered obese. The term "overweight" means being at a weight that is higher than what is set for your height and bone structure. "Obesity," on the other hand, is a medical condition. It describes someone who is eighty pounds or more over a healthy weight range, and has accumulated so much extra fat that it is health-damaging.

Chronic inflammation couldn't be more different from a classic case of acute inflammation. Rather than stemming directly from a known stimulus (like an injury) and existing in a specific spot, chronic inflammation develops over time and *slowwwly* starts affecting your body internally—often with few or no symptoms. Many people don't know they are suffering from chronic inflammation until months or even years after its initial onset! And once they do start feeling the pain or seeing other effects, they still might not connect that to inflammation, so they do nothing to reverse it and the inflammation intensifies.

If acute inflammation is a flash fire that roars into action and extinguishes quickly in a specific area, then chronic inflammation is a slow-burning, uncontained fire that can spread and destroy your body over months and years. For this reason, it has developed a reputation as a deep-state killer.

ARE YOUR DIET AND LIFESTYLE CAUSING CHRONIC INFLAMMATION?

There are many clues your body may be giving you to let you know it's inflamed. Take this brief quiz to find out. For each statement below, circle "yes" or "no."

1. You eat sugary foods such as candy, sweets, cookies, cakes, or soft drinks almost every day.

   Yes   No

2. You feel stressed out a lot of the time.

   Yes   No

3. You usually drink fewer than six glasses of pure water daily.

   Yes   No

4. Your meals rarely contain vegetables and fruits.

Yes   No

5. You have a fairly steady diet of fried foods, fast food, and cured meats (like hot dogs or lunch meat), eating them several times a week.

Yes   No

6. You easily catch colds or whatever "bugs" make their rounds in your office or home.

Yes   No

7. You have trouble sleeping at least three times a week.

Yes   No

8. You smoke or vape.

Yes   No

9. You rarely exercise.

Yes   No

10. You feel tired even after clocking ample hours of sleep.

Yes   No

11. You drink one or two alcoholic beverages almost every day.

Yes   No

12. You know you're overweight and need to shed pounds.

Yes   No

13. You tend to carry weight around your waist.

Yes   No

(continued)

14. You often feel aches and pains in your joints.

    Yes   No

15. You have digestive problems such as bloating, gas, constipation, or diarrhea.

    Yes   No

16. You have skin problems like eczema, or your skin is red and blotchy.

    Yes   No

17. You often develop bags under your eyes.

    Yes   No

18. You have an allergic or sensitivity condition that flares up for no apparent reason.

    Yes   No

19. You consume dairy foods such as cheese or milk almost daily.

    Yes   No

20. You use a lot of artificial sweeteners in your foods, and/or eat "diet" foods regularly that are artificially sweetened.

    Yes   No

ANALYZE YOUR RESULTS

This quiz isn't meant to diagnose chronic inflammation, but only to make you aware of factors that can cause it and pinpoint where your biggest issues might lie. Look over your responses. If you answered "yes" to several statements, you might be doing your body more harm than good. If even a single "yes" rings true and you don't have either a diagnosis or a logical explanation for it, you might be triggering chronic inflammation. At the very least, any "yes" answer red-flags habits or situations you can change. On a positive note, give yourself a thumbs-up for all your "no" responses; keep up the good work!

Inflammation and Your Fat Cells

Here's where things get really interesting and provide clues as to why you have trouble losing weight and keeping it off. Chronic inflammation can seep throughout the body, creating an environment ripe for weight gain. This situation can be caused by eating inflammatory foods, including sugar, refined carbohydrates, unhealthy fats, and foods to which your body is sensitive.

As we discussed earlier, inflammatory foods and the components in them cause your fat cells to swell up. They become sick and start acting like they're infected. They don't receive normal blood flow, and they stop releasing fat. Your fat cells get inflamed, big time.

As inflammation rages in your fat cells, they produce abnormal amounts of different hormones. Higher-than-normal amounts of hormones create even more inflammation, slow down metabolism, and make you vulnerable to disease.

Think of hormones like one of your favorite recipes. If you dump too much or too little of any one ingredient in the mix, this affects the outcome. Some hormone levels fluctuate throughout your lifetime as the result of aging, but other swings occur when your endocrine glands mess up the recipe.

Fortunately, you can control unbalanced hormones naturally, mostly with proper diet. Here is a rundown of key hormones and how they are affected by inflammation:

INSULIN. This hormone "unlocks" your body's cell doors to let blood sugar inside to be used for energy. Inflamed fat cells, however, create "insulin resistance"—a condition in which cells disregard signals from insulin and don't allow it inside their walls. Insulin resistance can lead to weight gain, an accumulation of belly fat, and type 2 diabetes. Eating clean, healthy, whole foods in the proper combination and avoiding junk food prevent insulin problems. So does including omega-3 fats from fish in your diet.

LEPTIN. Normally, this hormone transmits a simple message to the brain: "You're full, stop eating." As your fat cells get larger and more inflamed, your body becomes less sensitive to leptin's message. You go around hungry, wanting to raid your fridge all day long. Selecting anti-inflammatory foods, such as those on Power Plates, is a great defense against a leptin imbalance.

ADIPONECTIN. Often called the "anti-obesity hormone," adiponectin helps you burn fat, reduces your appetite, assists your body in using insulin normally, and increases muscle energy from glucose. But inflamed fat cells, especially those in the belly, put the brakes on adiponectin production, and fat-burning slows to a crawl. Levels normalize when you minimize sugar and refined carbs, eat more non-starchy veggies and power proteins, and work out regularly.

CORTISOL. Referred to as the "stress hormone," cortisol is normally discharged in response to circumstances such as waking up in the morning, exercising, and short-term stresses (like traffic jams, arguments, or deadlines). Cortisol also helps regulate inflammation in the body.

Normally, cortisol rises and falls, but with our super-stressed, over-scheduled lifestyle, our bodies pump out cortisol almost constantly, which can really mess things up, including our weight. When cortisol hangs around all the time, inflammation can get out of control, right down to the level of the fat cell. Excess cortisol also mobilizes triglycerides from storage and relocates them to belly fat cells. Too much cortisol is not a good thing! Fortunately, exercising and avoiding sugar and refined carbs help keep cortisol in check.

A MEDICAL TEST FOR INFLAMMATION

Through blood testing, your doctor can measure your level of C-reactive protein (CRP), a marker for inflammation, to find out whether chronic inflammation might be harming your health.

CRP is produced by the liver and rises when your body is inflamed. The amount of CRP that is produced varies from person to person, depending on diet, lifestyle, and genetics. If you smoke or vape, have high blood pressure, are overweight, or don't exercise, your levels are likely to be high, putting you at risk for heart disease or stroke. If you are fit, lean, and active, chances are that your CRP levels are low.

The Centers for Disease Control and the American Heart Association developed the following ranges of CRP scores to determine the risk for heart disease:

- Low risk—less than 1 milligram per liter of blood
- Moderate risk—1 to 3 milligrams per liter
- High risk—more than 3 milligrams per liter (this suggests raging inflammation)

These categories are the current medical standard and are reported to you in the results of a blood test.

How We Eat Our Way to Inflamed Fat Cells

Clearly, we want to stop inflaming our fat cells and avoid chronic inflammation at all costs—because we want to feel and look like our best selves. With chronic inflammation, there's no single, direct cause like there is with acute inflammation; rather, there are many contributing factors.

Top on the list of those factors, however, is diet. Your diet has the most direct effect on inflammation. Certain foods can cause or exacerbate its symptoms. I put these in two categories: inflammatory foods and reactive foods.

Meet the Inflammatory Foods

SUGARY FOODS AND DRINKS

Most of the sugar we eat—whether it's in candy, soda, baked goods, or straight from the sugar bowl into our coffee or our cereal—started out as a "whole" or unrefined food. In a lot of cases, it began as either a tall fibrous grass called sugarcane or as good ol' corn. Then in the refining process, these plants are stripped of all the good stuff—all the fiber and many of the nutrients—and what is left is just the sugar.

Americans eat a lot of sugar! Imagine 150 bags of sugar from the grocery store stacked in your garage or living room. That's the equivalent of how much each of us eats annually, according to the USDA. Plus, Americans slam down an average of fifty-three gallons of sugar-laden soft drinks annually. I don't think it's a coincidence that so much obesity and type 2 diabetes have occurred concurrently with the huge increase in sugar consumption over the last couple of decades.

There are two kinds of sugar: natural and added. Natural sugar is found in fruits, certain vegetables, and milk, while added sugar is the evil ingredient in many processed foods, like baked goods and sweetened beverages. Both kinds hit that sweet spot when you have a sugar craving, but added sugar is infinitely more dangerous because the processed foods it's found in are full of other junk—like additives and sodium—and few nutrients. (These are perfect examples of "empty-calorie" foods.) Added sugar can be converted to blood sugar so quickly that it is almost guaranteed to spike your insulin level and throw your body into fat-storing mode.

Natural sugars are found in fruits, veggies, and whole grains. When you eat these foods, you're also getting some vitamins, fiber, and other nutrients. One orange, for example, provides all the vitamin C you need for the day as well as plenty of folate and fiber, so the eighty to ninety calories it contains are well worth it. Foods containing natural sugars are okay because they're buffered with fiber and other nutrients.

Added sugar (the kind food makers put into foods and the table sugar we add to foods) can greatly kindle inflammation in your body, too. It spews out little devils called cytokines that spread inflammation in the body. These inflame your fat cells, and indeed your entire body. But that's not all. Sugar also diminishes the ability of white blood cells to kill germs. This problem weakens your immune system and makes you more prone to colds, the flu, and other infectious diseases. So minimize added sugar and foods containing it as much as possible! This highly inflammatory substance is clearly a big reason why a lot of people gain weight, especially at the levels in which it is laced into our foods.

As for high fructose corn syrup (HFCS)—after years of debate and speculation, scientists have finally declared that it is slightly worse for you than added white sugar (technically known as sucrose). Sucrose is 50 percent glucose and 50 percent fructose, while HFCS is typically 45 percent glucose and 55 percent fructose. It doesn't seem like that much of a gap, right? Well, researchers in Denmark now feel that 5 percent makes a difference.

After carefully measuring the HFCS in sweetened soft drinks, the researchers found that those beverages resulted in significantly elevated fructose levels in the body—more than the sucrose-sweetened drinks. When fructose is jacked up in the body, levels of uric acid go up, too. This is bad. Uric acid drives inflammation and is implicated in high blood pressure. The results of this study don't tell us that sucrose is better than HFCS. Sucrose is still awful. It's just that HFCS is more awful.

In addition, consuming a lot of HFCS is believed to cause obesity, insulin resistance, type 2 diabetes, liver problems, cancer, and chronic kidney disease. HFCS also inflames cells that line your blood vessels, setting the stage for heart disease. Added sugar in any form is a substance that definitely "feeds" disease.

I'm on a roll here, so I've got to bring up another downfall of consuming added sugar: its addictive potential. The more sweet foods you eat, the more sweet foods you'll want to eat. Once you give in to those cravings, you're right back where you started.

As proof, substance-abuse researchers have performed brain scans on people who ate sugary foods. When the volunteers ate sugar, their brains responded by increasing the release of the neurotransmitter *dopamine*—the so-called reward chemical. The same response occurs in alcoholics or drug addicts when exposed to their drugs of choice. Sugar can truly hook some people, eliciting a brain reaction that makes them want more.

Because the health dangers of added sugar are now known, food manufacturers are required to disclose on the Nutrition Facts panel of packages how much of the sugar in their products is added sugar. Personally, I try to keep my added sugar below 5 grams a serving, and it mostly comes from my snacks.

Reality check: I don't expect you to never eat sugary stuff again. C'mon, I'm a peanut-butter M&Ms person myself, but I go easy on them. Simply ease back on sugar, sweets, and processed foods.

Common culprits: Soda, commercial juices, snack bars, candy, baked sweets, and coffee drinks.

Try these instead: Fresh fruit, sweet potatoes, or dark chocolate.

REFINED CARBOHYDRATES

These include foods with added sugars as well as those made with processed grains. Some people call them "white carbs." Your body breaks down refined carbs such as white bread, pasta, and processed cereals into blood sugar even faster than straight sugar. This increases your insulin levels and allows inflammation to thrive, increasing your risk for weight gain, insulin resistance, and possibly type 2 diabetes.

You can't see unhealthy insulin metabolism, so it isn't as cosmetically obvious as a muffin top, but don't let it get out of control. Keep insulin in line so that you can dodge diabetes and its complications. This is every bit as important as looking toned in your swimsuit. Diet is not always about the number on your scale!

Also, refined carbs are often more difficult to digest and can damage your digestive system. Here's why: These junky foods have been stripped of fiber, vitamins, and minerals—so they can't feed your good-guy gut bacteria (probiotics) with the nutrients they require to thrive. There are also bad-guy bacteria in your gut. They love to munch on sugar and refined carbs for food, and when they get it, they start multiplying and overpopulating your gut.

This increase in bad bacteria crowds out the beneficial bacteria, causing changes in the barrier of the intestine. With fewer beneficial bacteria along this barrier, its "permeability" is altered. This means the intestinal wall gets so weak and delicate that it leaks unwanted substances like bacteria, toxins, and undigested food particles into your bloodstream. This condition is known as leaky gut syndrome.

With a leaky gut, the body launches an inflammatory immune response targeting the substances that leak through the intestinal wall. Symptoms are different for everyone, but among the most common are constipation, bloating, gas, brain fog, joint pain, and headaches. Some people even start craving sugar. There's nothing redeemable about eating a refined-carb diet!

Common culprits: Store-bought bread products made from refined white flour, pizza, crackers, pasta, pretzels, flour tortillas, breakfast cereals, and bagels. The white flour in many of these foods is loaded with inflammatory substances that can cause pain and hurt your health.

Try these instead: Whole-wheat bread, Ezekiel bread, buckwheat, quinoa, millet, oatmeal, steel-cut oats, or cauliflower crust (Cali'flour is the best).

GRAIN-FED MEATS AND PROCESSED MEATS

Eating meat is not unhealthy. In fact, you can enjoy it on Power Plates. But meat from animals that have been fed grain such as corn or soy (rather than grass) is a source of inflammation. A lot of corn and soy are full of inflammatory omega-6 fatty acids, while meats are high in inflammatory saturated fats. Both types of fats trigger inflammation in fat tissue, according to multiple studies, and fat cells get bigger. When this happens, they release pro-inflammatory agents that promote even more inflammation throughout the body.

When livestock eat grain, the animals get sick more often because grain isn't part of their natural diet. They're given antibiotics (the same ones humans use), which then enter your diet, too. This is disturbing on so many different levels. It means the roast beef you're having for dinner has probably been soaking in a potent drug cocktail far longer than that marinade you dumped on it last night. Like I said, you're getting secondhand antibiotics. A lot of medical experts think that this may slowly build a tolerance to antibiotics in your body so that they're less effective when you actually need them.

Livestock are also injected with hormones to help them (and us—YIKES) gain weight faster. As a result, our bodies think they're in a constant state of attack due to ingesting the residue of these substances.

As for processed meats, I'm talking about bacon, hot dogs, lunch meats, and so forth. The question is: Are they good for you? They're probably not as bad as you think, especially when consumed rarely and in small amounts. But living on a steady diet of processed meat can increase your chances of having heart disease, diabetes, and stomach and colon cancer. And compared with other meats, processed meats contain more inflammatory substances—which is why you've got to go easy on them.

Common culprits: Non–grass fed meat, bacon, hot dogs, bologna, sausage, jerky, and lunch meat.

Try these instead: Grass-fed organic meat, with red meat intake limited to twice a week. I know organic foods are expensive, but do your best. If you can't go organic, limiting your intake of non-organic meat is the next best thing. Don't eat too many hot dogs or bologna sandwiches, either. You've got this!

ANYTHING THAT'S FRIED

Foods that are fried in vegetable oil, like your beloved fast-food French fries, contain high levels of super-inflammatory substances that can harm your health.

Okay, what about air-fried foods? This is a very good question. Air fryers are appliances that "fry" foods by circulating hot air around the food. They require less oil than traditional fried foods, making them generally healthier than their oil-soaked counterparts. Other pluses: air-fried foods are lower in fat, calories, and inflammatory substances.

One caution, however: Air frying produces high temperatures at a very fast rate. This makes it really easy to burn your food. And burned food can contain cancer-causing agents. My advice is to air-fry foods in moderation, not every day. They are still fried foods.

Common culprits: French fries, fried chicken, fish sticks, chicken tenders, and onion rings.

Try this instead: Baking, steaming, grilling, sautéing, or roasting.

DAIRY PRODUCTS

In some people, dairy foods can be inflammatory because they contain saturated fats. Additionally, studies with full-fat dairy show that it disrupts our gut bacteria and annihilates levels of good gut bacteria, which fight inflammation for us. And lastly, dairy is a trigger of lactose intolerance, a common food sensitivity.

Cow's milk is particularly bad. It's processed with added ingredients and preservatives that inflame the body. So is full-fat cheese, which is chock-full of saturated fat—a big cause of inflammation. Cheese lovers can still get their fix with lower-fat cheeses.

I often suggest that clients with joint aches, pains, and bloating try cutting out dairy foods to see what happens. I remember one client who did this and got relief from her joint pain. Then one day, she ate a cheeseburger, and whoops, the pain returned. There is a definite connection between inflammatory foods and inflammatory symptoms like joint pain.

One reason that dairy, especially milk, is inflammatory is that it's surprisingly high in sugar. Regardless of whether it's whole milk or low-fat milk, one cup contains about 12 grams of sugar. Sure, it's natural sugar—lactose—but too much sugar, regardless of where it comes from, is inflammatory. If you're drinking milk with every meal, all that sugar adds up. Also, some people are intolerant of lactose—it's reactive for them and creates inflammation. Cheese contains less lactose, but as I mentioned, it's loaded with saturated fat.

Then there is the issue of dairy hormones. Dairy cows are regularly injected with growth hormones to boost their milk production. Further, the cows are kept pregnant as much as possible (more than 300 days a year), also for the purpose of improving milk production. The longer a cow is pregnant, the more estrogen and other hormones are present in its milk.

The hormones in dairy foods are "obesogenic," which means they stimulate fat production in humans when we consume these foods. It's best for your health to switch to non-dairy milks and products. That way, you'll sidestep these negative health issues.

An occasional serving of plain Greek yogurt, however, can actually help decrease inflammation, thanks to its gut-healing probiotics.

Common culprits: Cow's milk, cheese, butter, and ice cream.

Try these instead: Unsweetened plant-based milks, like cashew milk and almond milk. You can get a lot of calcium (synonymous with dairy foods) from green leafy vegetables.

REFINED COOKING OILS

Vegetable oils such as soybean oil and corn oil have a high concentration of inflammation-triggering omega-6 fatty acids and a low concentration of anti-inflammatory omega-3 fatty acids. And unfortunately, vegetable oil is used in many common condiments and sauces.

Common culprits: Mayonnaise, store-bought salad dressings, crackers, bread, and potato chips.

Try these instead: Grapeseed oil, extra-virgin olive oil, coconut oil—all used sparingly. My go-to oil for sautéing foods such as salmon is grapeseed oil; it has a high smoke point, meaning you can heat it to a high temperature and not lose its beneficial nutrients. Extra-virgin olive oil has a lower smoke point and is best for salad dressings and other non-cooked uses. Coconut oil is good for moderate-heat roasting, drizzling over salads and veggies, and incorporating in baking. (More on healthy oils on page 83.)

ADDITIVES

Most processed foods are laced with additives to preserve their shelf life, or to add artificial flavor or color. The body treats additives as invaders and tries to defend against them—which is a good thing. But if the body is constantly trying to fight off these invaders, chronic inflammation rears up its nasty head.

Common culprits: Most processed and packaged foods.

Try this instead: Stick to natural, clean eating. Read labels. If you can't pronounce any of the ingredients in the food, don't eat it. And shop the perimeter of the grocery store, where the natural, unprocessed foods are located.

ARTIFICIAL SWEETENERS

Certain artificial sweeteners really irk me. As it does with additives, the body treats them as foreign substances—a reaction that triggers ongoing inflammation.

One nifty study found that three sweeteners—saccharin, sucralose, and aspartame—can promote "glucose intolerance," a marker for type 2 diabetes and increased risk for heart attacks. Fake sweeteners alter the huge colony of good bacteria in your gut to favor the harmful bacteria that trigger inflammation and increase the risk for these diseases.

Further, fake sweeteners cause many of the same reactions that regular sugar does, because the receptors on your tongue and in your stomach can't tell the difference between the two. Artificial sweeteners actually trick the brain into craving more sweets and more sugar and throw your blood sugar levels out of balance. Also, our bodies weren't designed to process chemicals and other artificial ingredients. When you ingest one, the body doesn't know exactly what to do with it. So it surrounds that mystery chemical with fat and tucks it away someplace you'd probably rather it not be. Even though the diet soda you sip doesn't technically hurt your calorie intake, it does you no favors.

Your body simply has a hard time handling substances with "artificial" in their name. I think they are a slow poison—chemicals we don't need in our bodies.

Common culprits: No-sugar-added products, no-calorie "diet" soft drinks, NutraSweet, Splenda, saccharin, aspartame, and AminoSweet.

Try these instead: Stevia, Swerve, agave, or honey (all used in moderation).

TOO MUCH ALCOHOL

No, I'm not a party pooper. I enjoy a little tequila on Saturday nights when my husband and I go dancing. But all of us should consider easing back on alcohol intake. I know sometimes you get home from work and the kids are crazy and you need to relax. But even a couple of glasses of wine can switch off fat-burning. The liver stops its job of burning fat to burn off the alcohol instead. When your body breaks down booze, it creates toxic by-products that can damage liver cells, promote inflammation, and weaken the immune system. Excess alcohol further disrupts the anti-inflammatory action in our guts. Two or three drinks a week should be your max. If you don't drink at all, you're ahead of the game!

Common culprits: Beer, wine, and liquors.

Try these instead: Water, sparkling water, mocktails, or maybe just scale back by having one alcoholic drink or beet juice and tequila once a week. (More on alcohol on page 62.)

Meet the Reactive Foods

You might be allergic or intolerant to certain foods or ingredients in those foods. If so, these foods can trigger an inflammatory reaction in your body—which is why they are termed "reactive foods."

Reactive foods can be quite different from the inflammatory foods I just mentioned. In fact, reactive foods might even be anti-inflammatory! Remember when I mentioned I'm sensitive to onions? Well, onions in most people are inflammation fighters. Perfectly healthy foods can be reactive and trigger inflammation. It all has to do with your personal body chemistry. But if a food makes you feel unwell, that food is probably reactive to you.

What should you do? Fortunately, you can soothe the inflammation caused by reactive foods by cutting these foods from your diet completely, or at least easing back on them.

Food Intolerances Versus
Food Allergies

Food sensitivities include food allergies and food intolerances. It's important to note that a "food intolerance" is different from a food allergy. The difference is that a food allergy is related to your immune system, whereas a food intolerance affects your digestive system. Many more people have food intolerances than have food allergies.

When you're allergic to a food, it means that when you eat it, your immune system misidentifies it as a dangerous invader and sends out antibodies to fight it off. You suffer allergic symptoms as a result of the battle between the allergen and the immune system.

On the other hand, if you have a food intolerance, your body has trouble digesting the offending food, particularly the proteins in that food. Some food intolerances are caused by the lack of a particular enzyme. A good example is lactose intolerance, in which someone lacks the enzyme lactase required to break down lactose, a sugar in milk and other dairy foods.

With a food intolerance, your body simply can't digest the food well, and this results in many different types of negative symptoms such as bloating, gas, constipation, headache, or coughing. The symptoms of a food allergy are more severe than those of a food intolerance. For a small number of people, avoiding foods like peanuts or shellfish can be a matter of life and death.

It's a serious problem when people unknowingly eat foods to which they are reactive—and do so several times a day. This means every time that food enters the body, the inflammation starts its rampage. Without diagnosis or awareness, the damage is repeated over and over, meal after meal. The only way to get out of this vicious circle is by identifying the foods that instigate reactions and then eliminating them from your diet.

The chart opposite lists some of the most offending foods. However,

I must emphasize that they will NOT all be issues for you specifically. A food that is healthy for me may trigger inflammation and unpleasant reactions in you, and vice versa! The key is to identify which of these potential food triggers are reactive for YOU so that you can adjust your diet, burn fat, and transform your health and energy as a result.

COMMON FOOD INTOLERANCES AND ALLERGIES

OFFENDING FOOD	CAUSE	SYMPTOMS (These can vary from person to person and may not indicate a food sensitivity. Discuss symptoms with your physician.)
Additives and preservatives in foods	Nitrates/nitrites, histamines, MSG, sulfites, benzoates, and artificial colors	Skin reactions, breathing problems, digestive issues, pain of various types, swelling, among others
Corn, corn flour, corn starch, and corn syrup (Don't be afraid of corn kernels, unless you know you are allergic to corn. I love to put a little corn on my salads. A little bit causes no problems.)	Prolamins (zeins)—allergens that closely resemble the gluten proteins in wheat and cause many of the same problems	Fatigue, brain fog, bloating, irritable bowel symptoms, headaches, and joint pain
Dairy foods (These foods might not be a problem for you, but they are very reactive for some people and cause bloating.)	Lack of the enzyme lactase, resulting in lactose intolerance	Stomach pain, bloating, diarrhea, gas, or nausea

(continued)

OFFENDING FOOD	CAUSE	SYMPTOMS (These can vary from person to person and may not indicate a food sensitivity. Discuss symptoms with your physician.)
Eggs (I'm thankful I'm not sensitive to eggs, because I eat a lot of them every week.)	Various allergenic proteins	Itchy skin, nausea, and bloating
Fish	The muscle (flesh) and collagen found in the skin and bones	Hives, skin rash, digestive problems, stuffy or runny nose, sneezing, headaches, even life-threatening reactions
Peanuts	Various allergenic proteins	Hives, red skin, swelling around the lips and face, wheezing, coughing, throat tightening, stomach problems, irregular heartbeat, even life-threatening reactions
Shellfish	Various allergenic proteins	Hives, itchy skin, facial swelling, wheezing or difficult breathing, digestive problems, dizziness or fainting, or life-threatening reactions
Soy	Soy protein	Headaches, joint pain, acne, or eczema
Tree nuts— especially almonds, cashews, and pistachios— these can be life-threatening in susceptible people	Various allergenic proteins	Digestive upset, eczema, joint pain, and fatigue

OFFENDING FOOD	CAUSE	SYMPTOMS (These can vary from person to person and may not indicate a food sensitivity. Discuss symptoms with your physician.)
Wheat, barley, rye, and triticale, and foods containing them (I'm very sensitive to these foods and have to avoid them like crazy.)	Gluten	Bloating, tummy pain, diarrhea or constipation, headaches, fatigue, joint discomfort, skin rash, depression or anxiety, anemia

Real-Life Solutions

Over the past few years, I've been working with many clients who suffer from chronic inflammation, and the weight and health problems it brings on. I've helped them manage their diabetes, rheumatoid arthritis, celiac disease, and multiple sclerosis. These diseases are painful. They can bring you down. And too often, they're not diagnosed or treated, so they worsen over time.

To be clear: I'm not a doctor or a medical scientist. I can't diagnose you or promise to cure every ailment you're experiencing. But I am a National Exercise and Sports Trainers Association (NESTA)–certified nutrition coach, an elite personal trainer with more than twenty years of experience, and a front-row audience member to some absolutely *incredible* physical transformations. Many of these have come about when I helped people address their food sensitivities to learn if they are a reason for their weight issues and other conditions. This has been an important part of my nutrition and training business. The results have been remarkable. A few specific examples:

Karen lost fifty pounds after eliminating five foods that were reactive for her: wheat, dairy, nuts, sugar, and potatoes. Also, her Hashimoto's disease (a condition in which your immune system attacks your thyroid) went into complete remission.

After staying away from eating garlic and sesame seeds for two weeks, not only did Mary stop bloating, but also her joints didn't hurt, she wasn't hungry, and her energy was back.

Denise discovered that she was sensitive to corn, almonds, raspberries, and squash. She told me, "I removed them and felt like I had shrunk. Also, after many years of infertility, I became pregnant within three months of removing these foods." For the record, I'm not saying that eliminating reactive foods cure infertility or anything else. This was Denise's unique situation. What I am saying is that when you reduce chronic inflammation, your body can quit fighting unnecessarily and become healthier.

Sherry suffered from eczema, fatigue, bloat, digestive issues, and unexplained weight gain. It turned out that she was sensitive to wheat, bell peppers, dates, and pine nuts. She eliminated them from her diet and now feels like a new person: lighter, energetic, and healthy—and with clear skin.

These awesome responses are not unusual. I've seen dramatic effects in weight loss, overall health, and even mood and behavioral disorders when my clients identify and address their food sensitivities.

So how do you do that? Get a reliable test. Without one, it is almost impossible to identify which foods or drinks are reactive to you. Testing is vital to figuring out what exactly is bothering you. You can't just guess your way out of this!

There are a variety of tests for food allergies and intolerances. Two of the most common are skin prick tests and blood tests. In a skin prick test, a tiny bit of the suspected food is placed on the skin of your forearm or back. A doctor or another health professional then pricks your skin with a needle to let a bit of the substance get beneath the skin's surface. If you're allergic to that substance, you'll have a reaction like a raised bump.

A blood test can measure your response to particular foods by detecting the allergy-related antibody known as immunoglobulin E (IgE), which is associated mainly with allergic reactions. The presence of IgE antibodies generally indicates a food allergy.

Food sensitivity tests, on the other hand, typically look for the presence of immunoglobulin G (IgG), the most abundant type of antibody.

Some of these tests can only be ordered by licensed health-care providers (including medical doctors and dietitians) and others can be ordered online and sent directly to your home. Once you receive the kit, you follow the user-friendly guide and a simple, single finger prick is all that is needed. You send off your sample to a lab, and you typically receive your results, usually by e-mail, in seven to ten days.

Eliminating the reactive foods from your diet and replacing them with nutrient-rich alternatives helps resolve the inflammation and alleviates the negative symptoms. If you're overweight, or if you suffer from an inflammatory disease, such as heart disease or diabetes, the huge health benefits of discovering and rooting out hidden food sensitivities can't be overstated. Food is truly your best friend in helping you become the healthiest and most fit version of yourself.

Every time you eat, you are choosing to either fight or fuel inflammation right down to the level of your fat cells. The diet and lifestyle changes you'll make with Power Plates can really help get your body geared for fat-burning, easier weight loss, and awesome health.

3

CLEAN EATING

The Power Plate Diet is "clean" eating.

What do I mean by that? At its core, clean eating is making a conscious effort to eat as many unprocessed foods as possible and as few processed foods as possible. Clean foods (which are also called whole foods or natural foods) are unrefined and minimally processed—think fruits, vegetables, eggs, beans, lean meats, whole grains, nuts, and seeds. Super-important: Clean foods are anti-inflammatory foods.

Can you find it in the wild, buy it without packaging, or eat it without processing it in any way? These are all signs it's a clean food. An example of a 100 percent clean meal would be a spinach salad with grilled chicken, quinoa, avocado slices, strawberries, walnuts, and some olive oil. When you're consuming whole foods like these, you're powering your body with the most high-quality, inflammation-fighting fuel around.

On the other hand, most processed foods come in a box, bag, can, or other form of packaging; they've been altered in some way along their journey to the grocery store shelf. Although they're often more convenient than clean foods, the additives they contain can be dangerous to your health. When you eat mostly processed foods, you're polluting your body with *dirty,* chemical-filled stuff—and that will inflame your body and catch up with you in the long run, if not sooner.

In certain cases, though, processing is a positive thing for foods. Pasteurization, for example, makes eggs and dairy products safe for consumption. Also, unsweetened frozen fruits and vegetables are fine; in fact they often contain more nutrients than fresh varieties because they are frozen at their peak.

Bottom line: Toss out the junky processed foods, stock up on the clean whole foods, and combine them into the perfect Power Plate. Once you get going, you'll begin to see incredible changes, not just in your body, but in your overall health, sometimes within days. You'll lose weight you swore you could never lose. Your tummy will be flat for the first time in years. You'll grow stronger and stronger in your workouts. And your energy will soar. I've even had several clients who got the green light from their doctors to cut back on their medications because they started eating power foods in fat-burning combinations.

Clean Food and Your Body

A clean diet prevents inflammation, promotes weight loss, guards against disease, and turns back the clock on aging. But sadly, many people aren't properly informed as to what constitutes an anti-inflammatory diet like Power Plates—or how to follow one. Others feel that if they don't have an inflammatory illness (say, asthma, allergies, or arthritis), an anti-inflammatory diet isn't for them.

Not true! An anti-inflammatory diet is not only the best diet to follow if you have an inflammatory condition, but it is also the best diet for preventing and fighting cancer, possibly reversing type 2 diabetes, and fending off heart disease. And hands down, it is the best diet to fight obesity. When you eat clean with the right food combinations, you have the ability to literally manifest fat-burning at the cellular level. Eating clean is all about stimulating fat-burning, while enjoying mouthwatering meals made from natural, wholesome, anti-inflammatory ingredients.

To help you do that, I've handpicked a long list of power foods that are extremely high in healing nutrients and deliver substantial anti-inflammatory and fat-burning benefits. You'll learn about them in the next chapter.

The connection between diet and inflammation is clear: Processed foods can cause inflammation—so cut back on eating them as much as you can. Certain clean foods can reverse inflammation—so eat lots of them!

My Four Clean Anti-Inflammatory Eating Habits

Habits are routines we do every day, usually without thinking too much about them: brushing our teeth, taking a shower, getting dressed for work, and heading off to our jobs on the usual highway. Habits are a big deal. They free up our brains to do more complex tasks like solving problems and making important decisions. But habits can be good or bad. Often the bad ones are hard to break. Trying to do it can be overwhelming. My solution for helping people form positive habits and break bad ones is to keep it simple.

That's why I've drilled down to just four nutritional anti-inflammatory habits, all easy to do and grounded in practicality. When you see the benefits of following these habits—fat loss, energy, confidence, and more—you'll be transformed. Here are the basics:

#1: CUT OUT STARCHES AT NIGHT WITH MY MODIFIED CARB FAST

Contrary to countless magazine articles or blog posts you've read over the years, carbohydrates are *not* evil—or even unhealthy, technically (unless they are highly refined). I always say they're just misunderstood! Starchy carbs like bread, potatoes, legumes, and cereal provide you with a blast of energy once they hit your bloodstream and are broken down into molecules of blood sugar. This is why breakfast is considered the most important meal of the day, and it's why you usually need to refuel around lunchtime. A breakfast balanced with healthy starches and lean protein will get you through to lunch; a lunch with clean starches and protein will get you through the afternoon.

Which brings me to dinner—this is where it gets tricky. When you don't use up enough of the blood sugar your body creates from a starchy meal, it can be converted into stored body fat. Consuming nutritious starches in the morning and early afternoon makes sense because you likely will continue to move around for at least several hours after each of those meals, thus burning them off. But most people don't exert much energy after dinnertime—these hours are reserved for low-key activities like doing the dishes, helping the kids with their homework, vegging on the couch, and getting ready for bed. (If you exercise in the evening, the energy you get from your clean afternoon snack will get you through your workout.) On the Power Plate Diet, you'll do what I call my Modified Carb Fast—no super-starchy carbs after 3 or 4 p.m., and not again until the following day's breakfast. In other words, you'll "fast" from certain high-starch carbs at dinner and overnight.

I didn't just create this type of fast because I've seen such amazing results with my clients. The science supports it. If you eat most of your carb calories earlier in the day, your body becomes more "insulin sensitive." This simply means that it's using insulin as it should, and the hormone isn't piling up in your bloodstream, causing fat gain or the inflammation it brings on.

Timing your carbs earlier in the day can even put your weight loss on autopilot. A weight-loss study in Spain observed that volunteers who ate most of their calories, including carbs, before 3 p.m. lost around five pounds over twenty weeks, while those who ate calories later in the day lost no weight. Five pounds might not seem like much, but the volunteers lost it without dieting or exercise.

Another study of seventy-four women involved twelve weeks of a calorie-restricted diet where 50 percent of their daily calories were consumed either in the morning or in the evening. At the end of twelve weeks, the morning group lost more weight and had greater improvements in insulin sensitivity than the evening group. ("Insulin sensitivity" meant that their bodies were processing insulin normally, using it to regulate blood sugar and cutting down on fat storage.)

Fuel up with high-quality starches in the morning and afternoon, then cut off your starch intake before dinner, except for certain vegetables that are lower in starch and Power Plate–approved for dinner (see pages 76–77).

Carb timing with my Modified Carb Fast is super-important if you want to stay lean and fit.

HOW TO DO IT: There's no magic time to stop eating starches, but I recommend around 3 or 4 p.m. Yes, this means you won't be eating pasta or pizza for dinner—but there are lots of work-arounds so you don't feel deprived! (See the table opposite.) You can eat delicious starches earlier in the day. For dinner, try a substitute, like spiralized vegetable noodles. In chapter 7, you'll find all kinds of recipes—breakfast, lunch, dinner, snacks, and more—to get you inspired. I've even found a cauliflower pizza crust that has 6 grams of carbs in the whole thing *and actually tastes good*—the Cali'flour brand.

POWER PLATE WORK-AROUNDS

Power Plate workarounds are food swaps—easy and surprisingly tasty ways to prepare clean food, while satisfying your cravings for sweets and starches. Although these swaps will taste slightly different, they are also kind to your waistline and entire body—a trade-off you'll love.

The following chart below features ideas on Power Plate swaps to get you started.

STARCHY CARB SWAPS FOR DINNER

INSTEAD OF	TRY
Pasta and rice	• spaghetti squash (squoodles)
	• zucchini noodles (zoodles)
	• shirataki noodles
	• shredded cabbage
	• cauliflower rice
Potatoes	• mashed cauliflower
	• mashed parsnips or turnips
	• mashed cauliflower combined with mashed parsnips

(continued)

INSTEAD OF	TRY
Bread and tortillas	• Lettuce leaves, collard leaves, kale leaves (with the rib removed), cabbage leaves, large hollowed-out dill pickles, and ♥ portobello mushrooms are all excellent swaps for bread, wraps, and tortillas.
	♥ Cali'flour flatbreads

♥ My personal favorites!

#2: CUT BACK ON ADDED SUGAR

As I mentioned earlier, added sugar is highly inflammatory—flat-out toxic, really—and over time, it can lead to weight gain, disrupt your blood sugar levels, and cause serious health conditions like heart disease. Luckily, for those of us with a sweet tooth (my doughnut-loving self included!), the solution is "less sugar," not "*no* sugar." Your body absolutely needs *some* sugar in order to function—because, like starch, sugar is a form of carbohydrate and supplies energy to your body.

HOW TO DO IT: It's *so* easy to take in several times the suggested daily amount of sugar without even realizing it, but simply shifting into a clean eating lifestyle will automatically remove much of the added sugar from your diet. So whenever possible, opt for foods with natural sugars, like fruit, or a little maple syrup, agave nectar, or honey, and try to eat them earlier in the day so that you have time to burn off the energy they provide. Don't forget to keep your portions in check. Portion control is a MUST.

Zero-calorie sweeteners such as stevia, Truvia, or Swerve are also good options.

LABEL READING: HOW TO TELL IF A FOOD IS HIGH IN SUGAR

In packaged and processed foods, sugar comes disguised under different names. Look at the ingredients list on food labels and watch out for the following words—they're code for added sugar.

Barley malt	Fruit juice concentrates
Beet sugar	Galactose
Brown sugar	Glucose
Buttered syrup	Glucose solids
Cane crystals	Golden sugar
Cane juice crystals	Golden syrup
Cane sugar	Granulated sugar
Caramel	Grape sugar
Carob syrup	High-fructose corn syrup
Castor sugar	Invert sugar
Confectioner's sugar	Lactose
Corn sweetener	Malt syrup
Corn syrup	Maltodextrin
Corn syrup solids	Maltose
Crystalline fructose	Muscovado sugar
Date sugar	Raw sugar
Dextran	Refiner's syrup
Dextrose	Rice syrup
Diastase	Sorbitol
Diastatic malt	Sorghum syrup
Ethyl maltol	Sucrose
Evaporated cane juice	Syrup
Fructose	Treacle
Fruit juice	Turbinado sugar

#3: CUT BACK ON SODIUM

Even if you rarely utter the phrase "Can you pass the salt?" at the dinner table, you might be consuming too much sodium. That's because, along with its good friend sugar, sodium is literally baked into many processed foods that you know and love. Snacks, sauces, cheese, anything that comes in a can—they're full of sodium, sodium, and more sodium. Not paying attention to your sodium intake can lead to frustrating short-term issues like plateauing in your weight loss and even more serious conditions in the long run, like high blood pressure or heart disease.

Another big problem with excess sodium is that it can make you retain water. In the short term, you feel and look bloated and puffy everywhere from your cheeks to your ankles. (One of my sons describes it as the "Marshmallow Man" look.) Water retention is so discouraging. Those layers of puffiness hide all those pretty muscles you're creating through exercise, making your hard work seem futile.

Sodium overload in the diet also promotes tissue inflammation, joint swelling, and organ damage—all well-documented in research. So you really want to watch your sodium intake! Most Americans eat more than 3,400 milligrams of sodium daily—about a teaspoon and a half. That's more than double the American Heart Association's recommended limit of 1,500 to 2,000 milligrams.

I advise my clients to watch their sodium intake and keep it at or around 1,500 milligrams a day. This limited amount of sodium helps certain key processes in your body hum along smoothly, like your blood pressure, nerve function, and digestion.

How to do it:

- You're already reading food labels for added sugar, right? Check the labels for sodium and look for low-sodium foods (less than 140 milligrams per serving). After counting sodium for a few weeks, you'll get a sense of how much salt is in your foods, and you won't have to count it.

- Avoid processed foods and salty snacks as much as possible.
- Watch how much salt you add during cooking or afterward. A lot of sodium in our diets comes from adding it when we prepare food or when we salt it prior to eating. If you *must* add salt to a recipe, start with ⅛ teaspoon—you'll notice in my recipes in chapter 7 that this is my standard amount. I like to add salt afterward as opposed to while cooking food. I grind pink salt (my favorite); it gives a little crunch and a salty hit to my food. When you're cooking at home, experiment with herbs, spices, and low- or no-sodium seasonings to flavor your dishes. I can't encourage this kind of experimenting enough! I know firsthand, because salt used to be my weakness. It took me a long time to change my taste buds, but when they did adjust, I no longer needed to salt my foods so much. With less sodium in my body, I even got more defined and could see all the pretty muscles that I worked so hard to develop. Your taste for salt can change, too!
- Try a new seasoning on one of your favorite dishes, try a new dish with one of your favorite seasonings, and train your taste buds not to rely on salt for food to be tasty. Eating healthy with nutritious seasonings is never boring.
- Look for condiments marked "low sodium."
- At restaurants, opt for low-sodium items or request that salt not be added to your food.

 COMMON FOODS HIGH IN SODIUM

The foods I've listed on the following page are not all "bad"—you can enjoy them in moderation. Take bacon, for example. It sparkles up foods like roasted Brussels sprouts

(continued)

when you use it in tiny amounts. Condiments such as barbecue sauce are delicious and perfectly okay; just use them sparingly. And what would a taco be without some salsa? I just want you to be aware of foods that contain hidden salt.

Bagels

Baked goods

Barbecue sauce

Blended coffee drinks

Breads

Canned soups

Canned vegetables

Cereal

Cheese

Crackers

Cured meats

Dried beef

Fish sauce

Marinades

Olives

Pickles

Potato chips

Pretzels

Queso

Salad dressings (These are super-sneaky sources of sodium.)

Salsa

Salted nuts

Sauerkraut

Soy sauce (I don't use soy sauce anymore. I call it "liquid salt." I prefer coconut aminos—same flavor, but without the sodium hit.)

Spaghetti sauce

Tomato sauce

Tortilla chips

Worcestershire sauce

#4: CUT BACK ON ALCOHOL

Non-drinkers and rare drinkers, rejoice! You don't even have to think about the fourth and final clean eating habit—you're already there.

If you do tend to indulge, however, it's time to accept the fact that alcohol is not your friend. It's actually more like a frenemy, because on the surface it seems fun and cool and can make you feel good. But regular alcohol consumption can backstab you, eventually damaging your liver, heart, brain, pancreas, and immune system. And thanks to all those empty calories, especially in wine and beer, it often causes you to gain weight.

Too much alcohol also damages your intestinal lining. This damage causes harmful bacteria to leak into the bloodstream (leaky gut syndrome), triggering inflammation.

(To those of you protesting that red wine contains antioxidants and can lower your risk of heart disease: So can clean, nutrient-dense foods like berries, beets, and kale. And those won't destroy your body.)

I tell my clients to really start paying attention to how much they're drinking, meaning not only how often and how many drinks per occasion, but also how many actual servings of each drink they're downing. When you pour yourself "a glass" of wine at home, is it 5 ounces? That's one-fifth of a standard 750-milliliter bottle. From my "observational research," most people's pours are much larger—and that adds up. Moderation is key: Cut *back,* not cut *out.*

HOW TO DO IT: To drink wisely, a little strategizing can go a long way. Treat yourself to two or three drinks per week, max, and stick with it by planning out which nights you'll have a drink—and how many—so you won't be tempted when a friend wants to order another round.

Try not to drink alone. It's more satisfying to enjoy a glass of wine with a friend than to drink at home by yourself.

If water isn't satisfying enough on your non-drinking outings, explore the delicious world of mocktails. Club soda with agave, blueberries, and a splash of lemon tastes even better than a tequila shot—and you won't need to lick salt off your hand afterward, either.

Clean eating on Power Plates isn't restrictive. There is lots of room for flexibility and diversions, and it doesn't require cutting out any certain food groups—unless your doctor says so, or you're reactive to certain foods. The Power Plate Diet is meant to be a lifelong plan—one that's easy to enjoy forever.

After you commit, you should begin to *feel* better and more energized within days because you're getting rid of inflammation. Keep going because the process is so worth it. You're about to discover how great your body was designed to look and feel!

Now let's look at everything you get to eat on this plan.

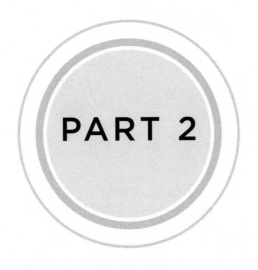

PART 2

INTRODUCING POWER PLATES

4

TORCH FAT WITH
POWER FOODS

The first question my clients usually ask me is: "What do I get to eat on the Power Plate Diet?"

I explain that they're about to enjoy the most delicious weight-loss-friendly foods on the planet—foods that will have big effects on their health and quality of life. With these wonderful foods, you coax the body into burning fat, prevent inflammation, and rev up your metabolism.

Exciting, right? You won't even feel like you're on a diet, while shedding pounds and inches almost effortlessly. You won't have to eat special foods. You can eat at restaurants. You can sit down with your family to comforting, satisfying meals. Within reason, nothing is off limits— even an occasional glass of wine. Once you follow my simple food guidelines and adopt my four clean eating habits, you can enjoy your life and get healthy and fit in the process.

Let's turn to all the specific foods your body needs to lose weight, stay energized, and resist inflammation.

Power Proteins

If ever there was a fat-proofing food, it's protein, the basic building block of our bodies. Protein:

- Takes more energy to digest than carbs or fat do. This means your body automatically burns calories after you eat protein.
- Helps you develop and preserve lean muscle from exercising. The more lean muscle you have, the more efficient your metabolism, and the more calories you burn at rest.
- Keeps your blood sugar in check, so your body doesn't produce too much fat-forming insulin.
- Supports the action of your thyroid gland for a healthy metabolism. One of the main jobs of your thyroid is to regulate metabolism.
- Acts as a natural appetite suppressant. Protein is filling! It curbs your appetite so that you don't overeat.
- Provides anti-inflammatory substances and amino acids such as taurine that protect fat cells so that they can adequately release fat.

Here are all the proteins you can enjoy on Power Plates.

FISH AND SHELLFISH

Packed with lean protein, fish is one of the best sources of omega-3 fatty acids, and is loaded with many nutrients, including vitamin D. Most forms of seafood are naturally tender and easy to digest.

Fish is also a must-have for fat-burning. Studies have shown that as part of a weight-loss diet, fish and fish oil can help you shed pounds and inches. A group of researchers from Spain, Portugal, Iceland, and the Netherlands observed that when fish was included in a weight-reduction diet, it promoted weight loss compared with diets without fish. This may be due to the fact that fish is an excellent source of fat-burning protein and inflammation-fighting omega-3s. It also appears that the more often you eat fish, the easier it is to lose weight. The reason for this may be the amino acid taurine in fish protein. Also, the omega-3s help burn fat, even belly fat.

Fish is just so healthy anyway. People in countries surrounding the Mediterranean Sea eat a lot of fish and have historically been known as some of the healthiest, fittest, and longest-lived people in the world. Of course, you don't have to move to Italy, Greece, or the south of France to make fish a part of your diet (but wouldn't that be fun?). For a taste of the Mediterranean lifestyle, I've got several flavorful recipes to incorporate fish into your diet.

Also, you get to eat different types of fish on Power Plates to keep things interesting. They all have different textures and flavors, and in cooking them, you can make them taste any way you want.

Anchovies	♥ Salmon
Cod	Sardines
Flounder	Scallops
Halibut	Sea Bass
Mackerel	Shrimp
Mahi	Trout
Mussels	Tuna, including ahi tuna
Oysters	

♥ My favorite fish

POULTRY

Poultry, especially the chicken breast, has become the go-to protein upon which many diets are built. But jeez, it can be boring. I mean, how many times have you found your mouth watering over a baked, unseasoned piece of chicken?

Never for me!

That's because I view chicken as a blank canvas to which I can add plenty of different herbs and spices. And it can be cooked in so many different ways—stuffed, baked, grilled, oven-fried, and more. Chicken and other poultry can be delicious and definitely not boring! Heed the words of a gal who has gobbled up her fair share of poultry (especially ground turkey, my favorite): Don't avoid it altogether, but do what you can to solve the boredom. Add it to any wrap, salad, sandwich, casserole, omelet, taco—or as a stand-alone, perked up with herbs and spices, and cooked in a healthy way.

If chicken or turkey are on your grocery list, it's healthier to choose poultry that's organic and free of antibiotics. Products like these make the food supply safer and keep you and your family healthy at the same time. Your choices really matter.

Eggs are "poultry," too. They're very versatile and can be used in lots of recipes. Eggs are weight-loss boosters. Two separate studies have found that compared with eating a bagel, having eggs in the morning can help you drop pounds—effortlessly, without even trying.

Yes, eggs are high in cholesterol, but recent clinical trials suggest they do not hike up your bad cholesterol or lead to heart problems or stroke, as previously believed. I eat a lot of eggs every week, and guess what? My latest blood work revealed perfect numbers in terms of cholesterol and other heart-risk markers.

Everyone is different, though. Medical experts are still investigating any links between eggs in the diet and conditions like diabetes and heart disease. If you love eggs, but are worried about cholesterol, use mostly egg whites.

That's what I do. I use a combination of eggs and egg whites in my recipes to keep them light. Egg whites are also more nutrient-dense than whole eggs—and they take on the flavor of whatever food you add them to.

Here are my recommended poultry selections:

Chicken, boneless, skinless

Eggs

Egg whites

♥ Turkey, boneless, skinless

♥ My current go-to favorite for poultry

RED MEAT

Red meat is good for you. It develops stronger muscles, creates healthier bones, and boosts the growth of brain cells. It really has no equal as a protein source, and has an amino-acid profile that's second to none.

With meats, I'm talking about beef, bison, lamb, and pork (which is technically a red meat despite being advertised as "the other white meat"). Beef and bison are tops. Besides the protein, B vitamins, iron, zinc, and other minerals, when trimmed of visible fat and cooked appropriately, they both deliver a saturated fat content similar to that of skinless chicken breast.

If you eat beef, choose cuts with "round" or "loin" in the name. These are the leanest because they come from the part of the animal that isn't as fatty. It's best to select meat that is between 90 and 95 percent lean to keep your saturated fat intake low. Check the package labeling for the percentage.

Pork center loin, pork tenderloin, and lamb tenderloin are low in saturated fat (the inflammatory kind). Most pork and lamb cuts have visible fat; trim this off prior to cooking.

Super-important: With any meat, go for those marked free-range, organic, or grass-fed, since other cuts contain antibiotics and hormones, both of which are toxic and inflammatory. I know that organic foods can be pricey. So don't worry if they're not in your budget all the time. Just do your best. Don't try to be perfect; try to be better. That's the Power Plates way.

Try the following, if you enjoy red meat:

Beef

Bison

Lamb

Pork

PLANT PROTEINS

If you don't eat animal foods and you want to shed pounds, you might be concerned whether you're consuming enough fat-burning protein. Not to worry: *All* plants contain protein in their whole form.

Plant-based proteins have some pluses over animal sources. They give you more fiber and less saturated fat, and they're also higher in a variety of nutrients. A diet containing a lot of plant foods can definitely help you lose weight, because they're high in fiber, and fiber keeps you full. So even if you're not a vegan or vegetarian, you may want to include plant-based proteins in your meals every so often.

My favorite sources of plant-based protein are *clean*—those that come straight from nature, compared with fake "meat" found in various food products. I can't emphasize enough, or in too many ways, that when you eat clean foods in their natural packages, you get all the nutrients they offer. You also eliminate excess salt and sugar, which can sabotage fat-burning.

Here are some plant-based proteins to consider when you're trying to lose weight:

Beans and legumes, all types

Edamame (young soybeans)

Lentils

Non-dairy milks and yogurts, unsweetened (almond, cashew, coconut, rice, or soy)

Nuts and seeds (these are classified as healthy fats, but are high in protein, too, and make great vegan protein choices)

Tempeh

Tofu

Vegan cheeses

Power Carbs

For years, we've been told to *eliminate* carbs if we want to get lean. The potato-chip kind, sure—but not the guys I've included on Power Plates.

"Clean" carbohydrates—those in their natural or minimally processed state—are incredibly important to your health. They're your body's main source of energy, and they're full of fiber and nutrients. When you eat clean carbs, they can actually help you achieve and maintain a healthy weight. Clean carbs:

- Energize your body for exercise to support fat-burning.
- Are loaded with fiber—a proven fat burner.
- Provide anti-inflammatory agents that protect the fat-releasing role of fat cells.
- Enable fat metabolism. Your metabolism is like a furnace. If you have a slow metabolism, your "furnace" is set on "low"; it's not burning very hot—which means it can't burn up all the fuel that you are putting into it. The fuel that doesn't get burned gets put into "reserve," meaning it gets stored as fat. If you have a fast metabolism, however, your furnace is set on "high"; it's burning extremely hot, quickly consuming all the fuel put into it, and burning excess fat. To run fast, your metabolism depends on stored carbs (glycogen). If there's little or no glycogen on

board, the body taps into your protein (aka your lean muscle) to manufacture glucose. So you're sacrificing precious muscle, and this can slow down your metabolism. It's better to energize your body—and your workouts—with some carbs than it is to force the body to eat its own muscle tissue for fuel.

Once I get my clients on clean carbs, they look, feel, and perform so much better. They find they have more energy throughout the day, and they can train harder in their workouts. And they get lean! Research backs me up on all this. A 2018 study in *Nutrients* found that overweight people who ate more carbs and fiber from clean carb sources lost weight and improved their body composition (they had more muscle and less body fat).

Another big plus for clean carbs—especially whole-grain foods: They can zap inflammation. Studies indicate that they reduce levels of C-reactive protein (CRP) in the blood—that marker of inflammation that I described earlier.

I know what you're thinking: What about the gluten in some whole grains?

I concede that some people genuinely need to avoid grains due to gluten-intolerance or celiac disease. This is a small population, however, and it doesn't mean the rest of us should throw out our whole-wheat pasta. Of course, if you're living the gluten-free lifestyle and it's working for you, there's no reason to change.

As with anything, you can go overboard on carbs, even the clean kind. If you do, this can stall your weight loss. And I'm not talking about going back to the days when you wolfed down a heaping plate of pasta with a few slabs of garlic bread. That's carb overkill. Instead, I mean eating in a balanced way that gives your body all the nutrients— including clean carbs—that it needs in order to perform at its best. Watch your portion sizes, and read labels to see what counts as a serving.

So say "yes" to moderate carbs! But stay away from them after 3 or 4 p.m. in order to help you get lean faster.

Here are your Power Plate carbs that come from the grain and cereal family:

*Amaranth

Barley

*Brown rice

*Buckwheat

Bulgur

Ezekiel bread

Farro

Kamut wheat

*Millet

*Oats (old-fashioned or steel cut)

Pastas (lentil and quinoa)

*Quinoa

Spelt

Wheat berries

Whole-wheat breads and tortillas

Whole-wheat pasta

* Gluten-free carbohydrate. (Oats, however, contain a trace of gluten.)

Power Produce
(Vegetables and Fruits)

Let's start with vegetables. If you haven't eaten vegetables since age five, we need to talk!

Avoiding veggies is a bad idea. Their health benefits are far ranging: weight control, energy (Popeye turned to spinach when he needed it), digestive health, heart protection, brain function, longevity, and more.

I loosely categorize vegetables into three types:

- Starchy veggies
- Low-starch starchy veggies
- Non-starchy veggies

The key distinction among all three lies in their total content of starch, a type of carbohydrate. It's often referred to as a complex carb, because it is made up of a number of joined sugar molecules. Starch is also found in a range of other foods, including breads, grains, cereals, noodles, and pasta.

*STARCHY VEGETABLES INCLUDE:

Arrowroot

Beans (kidney, navy, pinto, black, cannellini)

Cassava

Chickpeas

Corn, including air-popped popcorn

Green peas

Lentils

Potatoes

Sweet potatoes

Taro

Yams

* Do not eat these starches after 3 or 4 p.m. Enjoy them earlier in the day.

One large potato can contain more than 50 grams of starch, which your body will have difficulty using up in the evening. This doesn't mean you can't eat potatoes, but you should avoid them and other starchy carbs and vegetables in the evening.

As for low-starch starchy vegetables, they contain a significantly lower amount of starch per serving than those veggies listed above.

*LOW-STARCH STARCHY VEGETABLES INCLUDE:

Acorn squash

Butternut squash

Lima beans

Parsnips

Pumpkin

Spaghetti squash

Water chestnuts

*These options are fine to eat in the evening, as well as throughout the day.

The following group of non-starchy vegetables, which includes most flowering and leafy varieties, contains little to no starch—so dig in any time of day.

NON-STARCHY VEGETABLES INCLUDE:

Artichokes	Greens, all types
Arugula	Jicama
Asparagus	Kale
Bean sprouts	Kelp
Beets and beet greens	Leeks
Bok choy	Lettuce, all types
Broccoli	Mushrooms, all types
Brussels sprouts	Onions
Cabbage	Peppers, all varieties
Carrots	Radishes
Cauliflower	Shallots
Chard	Spinach
Cucumber	Summer squash
Eggplant	Tomato
Endive	Turnips
Green beans	Zucchini

All three categories of vegetables boast an impressive nutrient ré-sumé, with a variety of vitamins and minerals. Veggies are among the richest sources of heart-healthy potassium and magnesium. And they contain small amounts of other beneficial nutrients including blood-oxygenating iron and immune-supporting zinc.

Vegetables are also packed with health-protective antioxidants such as vitamins C and E and beta-carotene—all of which guard cells from damage. Antioxidants are believed to help fight the aging process and reduce your chances of getting chronic diseases like heart disease, can-cer, and diabetes.

It's no secret that all vegetables are high in fiber, which keeps your bowels moving. Lots of research suggests that fiber prevents diges-tive conditions such as inflammatory bowel disease, and reduces bad cholesterol, blood sugar levels, and the risk of heart disease. And since vegetables are naturally low in sugar and sodium, you can enjoy them without worries.

I want to mention that many starchy vegetables, especially beans and lentils, are good sources of protein. They contain up to 18 grams of pro-tein in just a cup. By comparison, three ounces of tuna yields 25 grams of protein. For this reason, beans and lentils are great swaps for meat in vegetarian and vegan diets. Their protein and fiber content promote feelings of fullness, too.

There are so many veggies from which to choose. . . . I'm sure you can find a few you like! Not only that, you can also do a lot to make eating vegetables a delicious experience: Sauté them in a little oil, add them to soups and stews, blend them into smoothies, or prepare them with herbs and spices, to list just a few suggestions. (See the sidebar op-posite for suggestions.)

Seriously, you will notice amazing changes in your body after eating more veggies!

GO WITH THE GREENS

Leafy greens are a favorite of mine for fat-proofing. First of all, they're rich in fiber. Fiber is a fat-fighter: It gives you a greater sensation of feeling full so that you're satisfied and not hungry. It also tends to lower circulating levels of insulin, a hormone that creates body fat and stimulates appetite. With fiber, your food is digested more slowly, and blood sugar enters your bloodstream at a slow, steady rate instead of one big spike. These actions help regulate insulin.

Second, greens are fat-burners. A number of studies suggest that eating just four cups of leafy greens a week can help you automatically shed five pounds in thirty days. Why? Leafy greens are not only incredibly nourishing but also very high in vitamins, antioxidants, and minerals, including calcium, which has been shown to stimulate fat-burning in some studies

My favorite greens are spinach, kale, chard, arugula, bok choy, collard greens, and dark green lettuces of all types.

NINE CREATIVE WAYS TO PUT MORE VEGGIES ON YOUR POWER PLATES

1. Toss them into homemade soups. As long as they are not store-bought, soups are a great way to eat multiple servings of vegetables all at once. For instance, you can puree tomatoes, cooked carrots, greens, onions, and other veggies into a soup base, along with herbs and spices. Adding extra veggies to soups helps to infuse your diet with anti-inflammatory goodness.

(continued)

2. Prepare veggie noodles. Easy veggie noodles are my favorite low-carb swaps for high-carb foods like white pasta. To make these "noodles," insert a vegetable—a zucchini, carrot, or sweet potato, for example—into a spiralizer. This handy gadget turns them into noodle-like shapes. It's as easy as sharpening a pencil. Serve the noodles just like pasta and top them with sauces, other vegetables, or meat.

3. Add veggies to sauces. Sneak veggies into marinara sauce, for example. Good candidates are greens, chopped onions, carrots, or bell peppers.

4. Learn to love cauliflower. Cauliflower is like the popular kid in school—everyone loves him or her. There are so many ways to serve it—mashed as a sub for mashed potatoes, riced as a sub for rice, and turned into a low-carb, gluten-free crust for pizza.

5. Blend veggies into smoothies. Toss fresh leafy greens into your smoothie, for example. Trust me, they don't compromise the flavor one bit, but are a terrific way to get more nutrients. In addition, frozen veggies, such as zucchini, pumpkin, beets, and sweet potatoes, work well in smoothies.

6. Enjoy a veggie omelet. Any type of veggie tastes great in omelets. My favorites are mushrooms, spinach, and tomatoes.

7. Try lettuce wraps. Use lettuce leaves as a wrap, or in place of tortillas, buns, or bread. You'll love my Lettuce Wrap Street Tacos on page 186.

8. Eat veggie burgers. These are a delicious and unique way to increase your veggie intake. They're typically made by combining veggies with eggs and other ingredients and placed inside a bun or lettuce wrap. (See my Beet and Bean Burger recipe on page 166.)

9. Try savory oatmeal. Oatmeal is typically enjoyed as a sweetened breakfast food, but you can make it a savory dish by adding eggs, herbs, and lots of vegetables. Check out my Savory Steel-Cut Oats with Fried Egg on page 153.

FRUITS

NOW FOR FRUIT: It is sometimes left out of diets. That's a shame, so on the Power Plate Diet, you get to eat fruit. Can I see a show of hands from everyone who approves? That's just about everyone in the room.

Fruit is nature's candy, packed with vitamins, antioxidants, and other anti-inflammatory nutrients that support a clean diet. Both fresh and frozen fruits are also high in fiber. Research has shown that if you eat fruit, you keep your weight in check and reduce your risk of diabetes, high blood pressure, cancer, and heart disease.

Fruit does have natural sugar in it, though, so don't eat three bananas or two cartons of blueberries in one sitting. I had a client who went on an all-fruit diet and gained seven pounds in one week!

I suggest that you treat all fruits like starchy carbohydrates and eat them early in the day, before 3 or 4 p.m. Watch your number of servings, and don't overindulge.

HERE ARE MY RECOMMENDED FRUITS:

Acai berries	Grapefruit
Apples	Grapes
Apricots	Guava
Avocados	Kiwi
Bananas	Lemons
Blueberries	Limes
Cantaloupe	Mangoes
Cherries	Oranges
Cranberries	Papaya
Currants	Peaches
Figs	Pineapple

Plantains   Raspberries

Plums   Strawberries

Prunes   Watermelon

Raisins

Power Fats

For too long, we've been fed the lie that an effective way to drop pounds is to stick to a low-fat diet. The logic goes something like this: Fat has more calories per gram than protein or carbs, so it stands to reason that, in order to lose fat, you should eat less of it, right? Not exactly.

Actually, eating fat can even help you burn fat! I know this sounds counterintuitive, but it's true. Fat improves levels of a fat-burning hormone called adiponectin. If you slash fat from your diet, this negatively impacts adiponectin. This hormone works to boost your metabolism and accelerate the rate at which fats are broken down.

Fat is also filling. When the fat you eat reaches your small intestine, it triggers the release of hormones CCK and PYY. Both hormones tell your body that you're full. The fuller you feel, the less likely that you'll nosh on fattening snacks or heap on a second helping.

With fats and oils, it's a good idea to exercise some quantity and quality control. They're yummy and easy to overeat, so I advise that you measure your fats and oils before using them. Drizzling a salad with oil can quickly escalate from a few teaspoons to several tablespoons, and one eyeballed spoonful of nuts might turn into the equivalent of three servings.

Here's a look at all the fats you get to eat on the Power Plate Diet.

NUTS, SEEDS, AND BUTTERS

Eating a variety of nuts and seeds in moderation may actually help you lose weight and feel full. The monounsaturated fat in nuts has also been shown to reduce inflammation. And seeds like chia, flax, and hemp provide heart-healthy, fat-burning omega-3s as well as protein.

You must closely watch your portion sizes with these foods. They are too easy to overeat. A tablespoon or two, or a small handful of nuts and seeds, is all you need daily. Keep nut butters to a level tablespoon or less.

Almond butter	Pecans
Almonds	Pine nuts
Cashews	Pistachios
Chia seeds	Pumpkin seeds
Flaxseeds	Sesame seeds
Hazelnuts	Sunflower seeds
Hemp seeds	Tahini
Peanut butter (natural)	Walnuts
Peanuts	

OILS

The top oils you should choose are listed on the following page. Olive oil contains oleocanthal, a molecule that has similar anti-inflammatory properties to ibuprofen, according to research. The highest grade olive oil is extra-virgin, and that should be your first choice. It is extracted from olives using only pressure (no heat), a process known as cold pressing. Cold pressing preserves the nutrients in the oil.

Macadamia nut oil is high in monounsaturated fat, which helps lower cholesterol. When purchasing this oil, look for expeller-pressed oil. It is extracted from the nut using a cold process so that all the nutrients are left in the oil.

Made by pressing the seeds of grapes, grapeseed oil is my favorite cooking oil. It is rich in vitamin E and a slew of anti-inflammatory natural chemicals. It's known as a heart-healthy oil, too.

Both safflower and sunflower oil are unsaturated fats, which are good to the body. They are loaded with omega-3 and omega-6 fatty acids, both of which can help lower cholesterol levels and cut your risk of heart disease and stroke. Sunflower oil has more heart-protective vitamin E than any other vegetable oil, including safflower oil.

I also love avocado oil. It has a light flavor and is very special because of its anti-inflammatory power. Numerous studies have found that this tasty oil may reduce the pain and stiffness associated with osteoarthritis. Avocado oil is highly versatile, too: It can be drizzled on food and salads, but it's also a safe and healthy cooking oil because its fatty acids stay stable at high heat.

Coconut oil is a plant-based saturated fat, but without the cholesterol-raising effects of animal-sourced saturated fats. It can actually raise your good HDL cholesterol. The beauty of coconut oil is that it is a fat-burner. It contains components known as medium-chain triglycerides (MCTs) that rev up the metabolism. Coconut oil also promotes feelings of fullness and has anti-inflammatory properties.

Avocado oil

Coconut oil

Extra-virgin olive oil

Grapeseed oil

Macadamia nut oil

Safflower oil

Sunflower oil

Power Herbs and Spices

When I talk to clients about clean eating, a lot of them say they don't like eating healthy foods because they taste boring. Do you feel the same? If so, that excuse ends in your spice rack.

There are so many different herbs and spices you can use to add kick to your meals. To make the most of your Power Plates cooking, keep a supply of fresh herbs on your windowsill or in your garden. Dried herbs, along with various spices, will work, too, when you want to perk up a bland dish without adding too much salt or oil.

Many herbs and spices have special anti-inflammatory benefits. Great in salsa, cilantro is a wonderful anti-inflammatory herb, for example. A research study showed that just twenty sprigs of cilantro a day helped decrease inflammatory markers in people with osteoarthritis. That's one powerful plant and one of my favorite flavors!

Then there's garlic. It contains a potent antioxidant called quercetin that fights inflammation in the body. When using garlic, smash it first and let it rest for a couple of minutes. This activates the anti-inflammatory compounds so you can reap the most benefits.

Ginger is a great herb to add to your diet, especially if you're suffering through inflammatory digestive issues such as ulcerative colitis and irritable bowel syndrome (IBS). Try sipping on ginger tea before or after meals, grating some into a smoothie, or adding some to your warm lemon water throughout the day. It's also a key ingredient in my beet juice (see page 194).

You may have heard of the anti-inflammatory benefits of turmeric. This root contains a compound known as curcumin, which is a powerful inflammation fighter. Turmeric can be added to many foods, including soups, curries, stews, and smoothies.

Herbs and spices are powerful, but they aren't magic bullets. If you eat a lot of inflammatory foods, you could have a turmeric or ginger or other-herb infusion, and it still wouldn't make a difference. It's better to combine them with other anti-inflammatory foods.

Here's a partial rundown of power herbs and spices I love:

Allspice	Moringa
Basil	Mustard
Bay leaf	Nutmeg
Chervil	Paprika
Chives	Parsley
Cilantro	Pepper
Cinnamon	Peppermint
Clove	Rosemary
Dill	Saffron
Garlic	Sage
Ginger	Tarragon
Marjoram	Thyme
Mint	Turmeric

Drink Water to Fat-Proof Your Body

One of the most important things you can do to fight inflammation and burn fat is also one of the easiest and cheapest: Keep your body hydrated. This is one of the first pieces of advice I give to all my clients, and there are many good reasons for it.

Your body's need for H_2O is more urgent than its need for any other substance except O_2—oxygen. Two or three days without water will put you at death's door.

This makes sense when you consider that our bodies are composed of 70 percent water. That water must be continuously replaced.

Alicia is a client of mine who started having dizzy spells, especially going up and down stairs and during her workouts with me. To look at her, she was the picture of health—slender and fit and busy in a high-level government job. But she could not shake the dizziness, despite going to multiple doctors. None of them could figure out what was wrong with her.

I was curious about her fluid intake. Alicia said she drank a lot of coffee throughout the day—that was pretty much it. It dawned on me that maybe she was dehydrated; after all, coffee is a diuretic and not the best hydration source. I suggested that she gradually increase her intake of pure water. A physical light switch went on in Alicia's body: As soon as she started properly hydrating, the dizzy spells vanished. Alicia had been suffering from dehydration, and the symptoms were scary.

Then there was my son Hayden, who is an excellent soccer player. He began having these weird dizzy spells on and off the field but would force himself through his games. Worried, we couldn't figure out what was going on with him. It turned out to be a case of dehydration. Hayden was not drinking enough water. Once I got him into the habit of hydrating, the problem was solved.

Ample water is clearly essential to health, weight, and overall well-being. First and foremost, it cools inflammation in the body by flushing toxins and other inflammatory irritants from cells. Water also helps lubricate your joints, which reduces joint pain and inflammation. And as you drink water throughout the day, your tummy will feel full, and you won't want to overeat. Adequate water is a natural appetite suppressant.

You need water to burn fat, too. The kidneys can't function properly without enough water. When they're not working up to par, they shift their workload over to the liver. One of the liver's main jobs is to metabolize stored fat into usable energy for the body. But if the liver has to pinch-hit for the kidneys, it can't get its own job done. Less fat is metabolized and unfortunately stays in storage.

Bloat is a sign you might not be drinking enough water. When your body doesn't get ample water, it perceives this as a threat to survival and holds on to every drop of H_2O. The result: water retention.

Clearly, the best way to resolve these issues is to stay hydrated. So how much water each day does that take? My general rule is to drink half your body weight in ounces of water daily. That means if you weigh 140 pounds, you'd shoot for 70 ounces, or just under 9 glasses. That would be your baseline. If you work out regularly (I hope so!), you need to drink water before, during, and after your exercise session. Hydrate more, too, if you are on medications or take in a lot of caffeine (both are dehydrating).

Do you have a "salt tooth" and eat a lot of salty foods? If so, you'll need some extra water to counterbalance the flood of sodium in your body. And keep your surrounding environment in mind: When it's hot and humid, or you're in a high altitude, you'll need extra hydration.

So drink up! Before long, you'll be the most healthy, fit person in the bathroom.

HOW TO DRINK MORE WATER

- Keep a full glass or bottle of water on your nightstand so that it's the first thing you see after you wake up. The body tends to be dehydrated in the morning. I recommend drinking 20 ounces of water as soon as you get up. Even if you don't feel dehydrated, your body needs to be replenished from the six to eight hours you've just spent sleeping. Can you imagine going that long without water during the day?
- Carry a full bottle of water with you all day long. Refill the bottle after you finish it. Also, there are special water bottles marked with ounces that help you keep an

eye on how much water you're drinking. These are a fun, visual way to measure your progress and encourage you to drink your quota.
- Don't like plain water? Jazz up the flavor with a natural enhancer like lemon, lime, cucumbers, or berries. Or infuse it with herbs such as mint, basil, or lavender. Experiment with various combos like lime and mint or basil and lemon.
- "Eat" your water. Many foods, including clean foods, consist largely of water: cucumbers, spinach, watermelon, grapefruit, tomatoes, grapes, and zucchini.
- Have one glass of water after you brush your teeth in the evening.

Along with regular exercise and my clean eating habits, eating these nutritious foods and drinking adequate water will pave your way to success, and a healthier life. Let's now turn the page and discover how to create Power Plates for every meal.

5

CREATE POUND-DROPPING MEALS

Planning your Power Plates is easy! It involves filling your plate with power foods for their anti-inflammatory and fat-burning benefits and satisfying your personal preferences. Most Americans plop too much meat and refined starches on their plates—a combination that just doesn't fuel the body optimally, and packs on fat pounds. They eat too few clean vegetables and too much inflammatory saturated fat.

So—how do you fill your plate without filling out your clothes? Instead of meat or refined carbs taking over most of your meal, you'll fill two-thirds of your plate with clean veggies and other plant foods. The remaining third goes to your power protein. Add a little healthy fat to the plate—and you create just the right fuel mix to fat-proof your body.

In this chapter, you'll gain a sense of what a Power Plate looks like at each meal and snack. Also, I've created lots of tasty recipes for you (see chapter 7). Each recipe serving automatically forms a Power Plate.

You don't need any special tools, except a standard dinner plate or tall glass (for smoothies) to keep your portions in check. Nor is any calorie or carb counting required. Just focus on filling your plate or glass with the right balance and portions of power foods. This is simple and works, whether you're eating at home or at a restaurant.

Let's get started.

Power Plate Breakfasts

A Power Plate breakfast jump-starts your metabolism. But if you skip breakfast, your body runs without fuel for many hours and will automatically store fat because it thinks it is in a starvation mode. Skipping breakfast is no way to fat-proof your body!

FILL YOUR PLATE WITH:

⅓ POWER PROTEINS

Fill ⅓ of your plate with eggs, egg whites, or a combination of eggs and whites; some lean turkey or chicken sausage; or Greek yogurt or a non-dairy yogurt. (See page 121 for a list of power proteins.)

⅓ POWER CARBS

Fill ⅓ of your plate with a whole-grain cereal such as oatmeal (placed in a small bowl) or a slice of whole-grain bread. (See page 122 for a list of power carbs.)

⅓ POWER PRODUCE (FRUITS OR NON-STARCHY VEGGIES)

Fill the remaining ⅓ of your plate with fruit, such as berries, banana slices, or apple slices. Alternatively, scramble your eggs or egg whites with non-starchy veggies such as greens, mushrooms, tomatoes, or onions. (See page 125 for a list of power fruits and page 124 for a list of power non-starchy veggies.)

Sample Power Plate Breakfasts

- Egg whites and oatmeal topped with fresh berries
- Almond milk yogurt topped with sliced bananas and a slice of whole-grain toast
- Egg white omelet with spinach, diced tomatoes, and chopped onions and a slice of whole-grain toast
- Any Power Plate breakfast recipe (beginning on page 137):
  - Avocado Toast on Ezekiel Bread with Eggs
  - Quinoa Porridge
  - Chia Seed Pudding
  - Sweet Plantain Waffles
  - Mashed Banana Oatmeal
  - Power Oats
  - Almond Flour Pancakes
  - Southwestern Breakfast Burrito
  - Egg Muffins with Whole-Grain Toast
  - Banana Cinnamon Pancakes
  - Breakfast Quiche with Sweet Potato Crust
  - Roasted Acorn Squash with Yogurt, Honey, and Nuts
  - Breakfast Casserole with Sweet Potatoes, Broccoli, and Peppers
  - Overnight Steel-Cut Oats
  - Acai Breakfast Bowl

Power Plates for Breakfast at a Restaurant

- Yogurt parfait (Greek yogurt, fresh fruit, and a little granola)
- Scrambled egg whites, slice of rye toast, and a small fruit bowl
- Scrambled eggs, bowl of oatmeal or grits, and a small fruit bowl
- Turkey sausage or turkey bacon, slice of whole-wheat toast, and a small fruit bowl
- Egg white omelet made with spinach, mushrooms, onions, tomato, and other veggies, slice of whole-wheat toast

- Smoked salmon, whole-grain English muffin, slice of red onion, and capers

Or, start your day with a smoothie. On super-busy days, I love to whip up a smoothie for breakfast. The same Power Plate formula applies. For example: a cup of unsweetened almond milk (power protein), a handful of raw oats (power carbs), and a handful of frozen berries or kale or both (power produce)—with a little honey or other sweetener.

Try the following smoothie recipes for breakfast:

Beets and Tart Cherry Smoothie

Creamy Avocado and Mint Smoothie

Pumpkin Protein Smoothie

Power Plate Lunches

Yes, breakfast is sometimes considered the most important meal of the day, but don't let lunch play second fiddle to other meals. Eating a Power Plate lunch stabilizes your blood sugar level so that your energy doesn't take a nosedive by midafternoon. A Power Plate lunch also boosts your concentration in the late afternoon, and it helps you avoid hunger and cravings that can lead to overindulging on the wrong foods or raiding the vending machine.

FILL YOUR PLATE WITH:

⅓ POWER PROTEINS

Fill ⅓ of your plate with poultry, fish, meat, or plant protein. (See page 121 for a list of power proteins.)

⅓ POWER CARBS OR STARCHY VEGETABLES

Fill ⅓ of your plate with a whole grain such as brown rice, quinoa, or whole-wheat pasta; or a starchy vegetable such as peas, corn, or a potato, or sweet potato; or a low-starch starchy vegetable like squash. (See page 122 for a list of power carbs.)

⅓ POWER PRODUCE (NON-STARCHY VEGGIES)

Fill the remaining ⅓ of your plate with non-starchy veggies, such as greens, asparagus, broccoli, cauliflower, beets, Brussels sprouts, zucchini, or salad vegetables. (See page 124 for a list of power veggies.)

Sample Power Plate Lunches

- Tuna atop a bed of greens and a side of brown rice, drizzled with a tablespoon of olive oil and a little balsamic vinegar
- Lean ground beef, cooked, with 2 whole-wheat tortillas, and diced tomatoes and jalapeños
- Roasted chicken breast, asparagus, and a baked potato
- Hummus served with 1 whole-wheat tortilla or pita bread with a sliced tomato
- A bowl made with quinoa, salmon, and your choice of non-starchy veggies
- A sandwich made with 2 slices of Ezekiel bread, baked chicken or turkey, avocado slices, and mustard; and a side salad, drizzled with a tablespoon of olive oil and a little balsamic vinegar
- Any Power Plate lunch recipe (beginning on page 151):
  - Spicy Lentil and Sweet Potato Salad with Vinaigrette
  - Quinoa Pasta with Pan-Seared Chicken and Creamy Avocado Spinach Sauce
  - Savory Steel-Cut Oats with Fried Egg
  - Roasted Butternut Squash Pecan Quinoa Salad

- Lentil Pasta with Butternut Squash "Cheesy" Sauce
- Barley Salad with Lemony Kale Pesto
- Quinoa, Tempeh, and Roasted Veggie Salad with Walnut Dressing
- Strawberry Spinach Salad with Tofu and Simple Dressing
- Creamy Avocado Chicken Salad Wraps
- Broiled Orange Teriyaki Salmon with Edamame and Quinoa
- Shredded Brussels Sprouts and Kale Salad with Roasted Sweet Potatoes and Almond Butter Dressing
- Quinoa-Stuffed Acorn Squash
- Tuna Salad Sandwich
- Healthy Egg Salad Wrap
- Beet and Bean Burger

Power Plates for Lunch at a Restaurant

- Grilled chicken atop a salad (drizzled with olive oil) and a baked sweet potato
- "Buddha bowl"—a bowl of various vegetables, legumes, and other plant protein such as tofu
- Any type of salad bowl containing a protein, veggies, quinoa (or other starch), and avocado or nuts
- Grilled chicken, beef burger, or bean burger on a whole-grain bun with a side salad
- Fresh greens with oil and vinegar dressing, topped by grilled shrimp, and a starch such as brown rice or quinoa on the side
- A sandwich wrap with grilled chicken or tuna, avocado, and veggies
- Hummus with cucumbers for dipping and whole-grain pita bread

Power Plate Dinners

Dinners consist only of power vegetables (including low-starch starchy veggies) and power proteins. Remember, you won't be eating starchy foods after 3 or 4 p.m. in order to accelerate your fat loss.

Design your dinner plate with brightly colored vegetables, choosing from green, red, orange, purple, and yellow veggies. Those with the brightest, deepest colors pack the most anti-inflammatory punch.

FILL YOUR PLATE WITH:

⅓ POWER PROTEINS

Fill ⅓ of your plate with poultry, fish, meat, or plant protein. (See page 121 for a list of power proteins.)

⅔ POWER PRODUCE (LOW AND NON-STARCHY VEGGIES)

Fill the remaining ⅔ of your plate with low-starch starchy veggies such as squash, parsnips, or lima beans; and non-starchy vegetables like greens, asparagus, broccoli, cauliflower, beets, Brussels sprouts, zucchini, or salad vegetables. (See page 124 for a list of power non-starchy veggies.)

Sample Power Plate Dinners

- Grilled salmon, parsnips, and broccoli
- Baked turkey breast, acorn squash, and spinach or kale
- Lean ground beef cooked in unsweetened pasta sauce atop spiralized zucchini (zoodles)
- Stir-fried vegetables with cauliflower rice and edamame
- Any Power Plate dinner recipe (beginning on page 169):
    - Honey Sesame Seared Salmon with Spicy Cabbage Slaw
    - Curry Chicken Lettuce Wraps

- Chicken Enchilada Cauliflower Rice Bowl
- Turkey Meatballs with Zucchini Noodles and Avocado Sauce
- Slow-Cooker Beef with Broccoli
- Pesto Whitefish Packets with Veggies
- Low-Carb Chicken Pad Thai with Vegetable Noodles
- Chicken Alfredo Spaghetti Squash
- Crunchy Coconut and Kale Salmon
- Chicken Zoodle Soup
- Cauliflower Crust BBQ Pizza
- Cauli-Fried Rice with Eggs and Veggies
- Steak Salad with Rosemary Olive Oil Dressing
- Lettuce Wrap Street Tacos
- Salmon and Scallops Salad
- Szechuan Eggplant
- Quick and Easy Black Bean Enchiladas
- Stuffed Poblano Peppers

Power Plates for Dinner at a Restaurant
- Grilled salmon with broccoli, or any fresh fish with seasonal vegetables and a garden salad with oil and vinegar dressing on the side
- Grilled chicken with steamed vegetables and salad with oil and vinegar dressing
- Sashimi and seaweed salad, a cucumber salad, or a simple house salad with oil and vinegar dressing
- Chicken cacciatore with spaghetti squash if available at an Italian restaurant
- Fajita chicken, beef, or shrimp—without the tortillas but wrapped in lettuce—with plenty of grilled veggies
- Filet mignon or small sirloin, vegetable medley, and tossed side salad with oil and vinegar dressing
- Large Ahi tuna appetizer and tossed side salad with oil and vinegar dressing

Power Plate Snacks and Treats

If you want the fat-burning fire to burn you've got to keep fueling it. One way to do that is to include two snacks daily in your meal planning. Believe it or not, skipping those snacks can actually slow your metabolism, not speed it up.

So add to your satisfaction with snacks—up to two snacks or treats a day—one at midmorning and the other in the midafternoon. Or have one snack during the day and add a treat for dessert at lunch or dinner. There are many different ways to create Power Plate snacks and treats. Enjoy these occasionally. Try the following:

- Fruit and a fat (apple slices with 1 tablespoon of almond butter, or a peach with a handful of almonds)
- A single piece of fresh fruit
- Raw power veggies and 2 tablespoons of hummus
- A smoothie
- A power carb (1 serving of air-popped popcorn, for example)
- Protein and fruit (a cup of almond yogurt with freshly sliced strawberries)
- Any of my Power Plate snack or treat recipes (beginning on page 191):
  - Peanut Butter Energy Balls
  - Black Bean Brownies
  - Healthy Banana Nut Bread
  - Banana Ice Cream
  - Protein Berry Muffins
  - Healthy Freezer Fudge
  - Banana Oatmeal Cookies
  - Dessert Pizza
  - Pumpkin Bars

- No-Bake Cheesecake Bites
- Tart Cherry Lime Gummies

Using Power Fats

Add power fats to any Power Plate in small amounts: slices of avocado on salads, 1 to 2 tablespoons of oil as salad dressing or to cook with, or a handful of nuts or seeds on veggies or as snacks. Treat fats as a condiment, and you can't go wrong.

12 POWER PLATE POINTERS FOR SUCCESS

1. Fuel your body. Power Plates fill up your energy tanks. In the correct balance and portions, eating three meals and two snacks daily helps avoid hunger that leads to temptation, plus energizes you for your workouts.
2. Focus on a variety of food choices. The greater the mix, the more nutrients you'll obtain.
3. Try new recipes weekly. Learning how to prepare new dishes will help you appreciate them more—and make it easier for you to stick to your Power Plates eating plan.
4. Be adventurous. Buy at least one new food—an exotic grain like quinoa or some plantains—every time you go grocery shopping. If you like it, incorporate it into your usual meal plans. If not, try something else next time.
5. Climb out of ruts. Veggies don't always have to be boiled; roast or stir-fry them. And don't just think white potatoes. Think Purple Passion potatoes, Yukon Golds, or sweet potatoes or yams.
6. Don't pile too much food on each segment of your

(continued)

plate. If food overflows the rim of your plate, you're probably going to eat more food than your body needs or can burn off. Power Plates give you automatic portion control.

7. Eat until you're satisfied, not stuffed. Eat slowly and enjoy the flavors, too.
8. Use anti-inflammatory herbs and spices liberally on your foods.
9. Consider going meatless a few meals each week and include plant-based proteins in your Power Plates.
10. Avoid foods that are reactive to you.
11. Stay hydrated.
12. Rely less on your scale. I'm not a "scale person." I'd rather you focus on the increased energy you have now, the way your skirt or pants no longer dig into your tummy, how easy it is to climb a flight of stairs, or the decrease in your blood pressure. The scale is not always your best measure of success.

Power Plates Diet Boosters

I recommend that you take two really important supplements on the Power Plate Diet: fresh beet juice (which isn't technically a supplement, but a natural food) and collagen peptide protein. I've researched both quite extensively and use them myself, so I know their power!

BEET JUICE

Beet juice changed my life in a month's time—mainly in powering up my body to unheard of levels of energy. Since I started taking beet juice, I saw major improvements in my stamina and athletic abilities. Beet juice reduced my run time by two to three minutes in two weeks and dropped my resting heart rate by ten digits.

Beet juice is an enormously powerful way to protect your health. A 2019 article in *Medical News Today* listed six health benefits. Beet juice:

1. Is high in antioxidants, vitamins, and minerals that improve cellular health, protect organs, strengthen immunity, and boost metabolism.
2. Reduces abnormal blood clotting and high blood pressure. Research from a large team of Australian investigators found that it protects arteries from pro-inflammatory substances that can lead to dangerous clotting and high blood pressure.
3. Reduces inflammation. Beet juice contains anti-inflammatory compounds called betalains, responsible for the deep red color of the beet. Betalains curtail the activity of enzymes that cause inflammation in the body. Beet juice is one of my favorite anti-inflammatory foods.
4. Prevents anemia. Beet juice is a strong source of iron, which is responsible for transporting oxygen around the body. Without iron, red blood cells don't get enough oxygen, and a condition called iron-deficient anemia is the result. I have sometimes struggled with this, so I make sure I drink beet juice consistently.
5. Protects the liver. Beet juice helps protect the liver from inflammation while enhancing its ability to eliminate toxins from the body (which can help fight overweight and obesity).
6. Boosts athletic performance. As proven in research, beet juice opens your blood vessels and allows more oxygen in. This oxygen-boosting action keeps you from getting winded.

Don't like the taste of beets? Here's how I convinced my family, friends, and clients to give it a try: My recipe (see page 194) requires only three ingredients—beets, ginger, and lemon—and tastes sort of like a zesty lemonade. The lemons take the flavor, the beets sweeten the lemons, and the ginger gives the whole thing a little kick. If it tasted bad, I wouldn't drink it every day and tell everyone I know to do the same. I've had *many* clients push back against the whole beet thing before actually trying it—but I haven't had a single one prove me wrong.

I take two three-ounce shots daily—one in the morning after breakfast and one late in the afternoon (usually an hour prior to my workout), and never on an empty stomach. You'll love it! I like to prep my beet juice in advance, and I make it for my whole family. Stored in a glass container, a whole batch lasts around three days, so drink it within that time frame. We juice it up a couple of times a week. A little goes a long way: Just a three-ounce shot is one serving. On Saturdays, I like to mix my second beet juice shot with tequila to make a unique, fun, and healthy mixed drink. My favorite!

I've tried store-bought beet juice, but honestly it doesn't work as well. Beet juice needs to be fresh. The heat used in pasteurization to make it shelf-stable destroys its benefits.

One caveat: If you've had kidney stones, beet juice can aggravate this condition.

COLLAGEN PEPTIDES

I also add one scoop of collagen peptide powder to my beet juice right before I take it. Collagen peptides are kind of magical. They're a tasteless, odorless powder that dissolves in nearly any food or liquid and improves the health of your joints, bones, hair, skin, and nails. You can add them to your shot of beet juice, your clean breakfast, your coffee—wherever it works best for you.

I only discovered this supplement a few years ago and wish I had known about it sooner. I had to have knee surgery because I tore my ACL playing soccer, and I tore my meniscus twice. Ever since the surgery, I've used collagen peptides for pain and recovery because of the improvements they've made in my joints. When I don't take collagen, I can really tell. But with them, I'm able to do all I want without pain.

Here's some background: Collagen is one of the most abundant proteins in the body. It is the structural component of our connective tissue, found in skin, bones, muscles, tendons, and ligaments. It works with another protein called elastin to keep the skin supple and healthy.

As we age, our bodies scale back on collagen production—which is why we need to take collagen peptide supplements. The peptides are tiny chains of protein that are easily absorbed into areas that need repair and rejuvenation the most. Made of bovine, poultry, and marine collagen, these supplements have been found in research to:

- Increase skin elasticity
- Prevent skin aging
- Reduce skin roughness
- Make nails grow faster (by about 12 percent)
- Support hair growth
- Reduce the occurrence of brittle nails and broken nails
- Improve joint health
- Promote gut health, which is also important for fighting inflammation
- Increase bone density in bones weakened with age.

Pretty amazing, right? I take two scoops every day and have seen remarkable results not only in my knees, but also in my hair, nails, and skin. Collagen is a true and effective elixir that should be taken for life to maintain healthy levels of collagen in your body. Follow the manufacturer's suggestion for dosage.

Collagen peptides are used in several of my recipes (see chapter 7). If you're vegetarian or vegan, omit the collagen peptides in these recipes, as the peptides are sourced from animals. Marine collagen is an option for pescatarians (it's usually sourced from snapper, cod, or salmon). Unfortunately, a vegetarian/vegan version doesn't exist yet.

WHAT ABOUT OTHER SUPPLEMENTS?

I'm often asked: "Should I be taking nutritional supplements?"

My answer, honestly, is: "It depends."

For some people, taking certain supplements may be the best way to get nutrients they are missing from their diets. For example, if you don't eat fish, you may need an omega-3 fatty acid supplement. Or you may need to supplement your diet if you have a medical condition in which your body does not properly absorb or use nutrients—or your doctor has determined you're deficient in certain nutrients. If pregnant, you may need a prenatal supplement. If you're a vegan or vegetarian who eats a limited variety of foods, supplementing may be warranted, especially with vitamin B_{12} (found in animal foods). Vegans and vegetarians sometimes don't get enough of this nutrient unless they supplement.

However, obtaining nutrients from clean foods is the best course of action, whenever possible. Supplements cannot replicate all the health benefits of whole foods. A red bell pepper, for instance, provides vitamin C, plus some beta-carotene, calcium, and other nutrients. In foods, nutrients like these work synergistically to produce a beneficial effect.

Clean foods are loaded with other nutrients important for good health. For example, power carbs and power produce contain naturally occurring antioxidants and anti-inflammatory substances that may help protect against cancer, cardiovascular disease, diabetes, and high blood pressure. And many clean foods, such as whole grains, vegetables, legumes, and fruit are packed with fiber. Fiber in food offers great protection against diseases such as diabetes and heart disease. It can also help manage constipation and fight weight gain.

It's important to understand what your exact needs are before getting out your wallet and buying every supplement in the vitamin store. But if you want to take supplements, that's fine. Everyone is different. We all should make decisions with our health-care providers based on our health, life, and individual situations.

Remember, the key to success on the Power Plate Diet is eating the right combinations of anti-inflammatory power foods in the right amounts. In the next chapter, I'll help you by providing sample daily menus for four entire weeks. You can follow them to the letter, or adapt them to your own preferences. The menus include my Power Plate recipes for breakfast, lunch, dinner, snacks, and treats (see chapter 7). I can't wait to show you these delicious menus and how to fit them into your fat-proofing way of life.

6

YOUR POWER PLATES FOUR-WEEK EATING PLAN

Now is the time to create your Power Plates so that you can reach your health and fitness goals—plus energize yourself for my workouts. Sure, you might be the rare person who can just wing it from meal to meal, but most of us need some structure for long-term success.

Here, you'll find my four-week Power Plates meal plan. This first month will get you accustomed to the Power Plates way of eating—and solidify nutritious habits. But remember: This isn't a "four weeks and you're fixed" plan. It's designed to be continued well past the four weeks and be a part of your lifestyle forever.

The plan also includes guidance on how to create your own plan using my diet principles. These principles take into account the four elements of a perfect anti-inflammatory Power Plate: clean proteins, carbohydrates at breakfast and lunch, vegetables, and healthy fats.

Here are a few important guidelines and tips, based on how I advise my clients to organize and customize their meal plans.

Be Flexible

I've learned that my clients want flexibility, nothing rigid. Some are fine with following a menu plan to the letter, recipes and all, while others are DIYers. They like to pick and choose from Power Plate–approved foods and organize their own meals. Still others like to do a little of both.

If you're a DIYer, follow the meal-planning principles described in the previous chapter. They show you how to divide and fill your plates at each major meal. Then refer to the food lists beginning on page 121 to select the foods you want on your plate.

If you'd rather follow a meal plan with recipes to the letter—without having to think—simply follow the four-week meal plan that begins on page 110. It gives you daily meals that are delicious, satisfying, and help you take off inches and pounds.

Maybe you're somewhere in between—you like to try new recipes but also enjoy the independence of planning your own meals. It's fine to include both DIY meals and meals with recipes. Also, it's perfectly fine to enjoy the same meals a few days in a row if you have favorites—the Power Plate Diet is super-flexible.

Consider Variety

When I first started developing my Power Plates diet, I wanted lots of variety. Someone could have a different breakfast, lunch, and dinner nearly every day. It sounded great, but following something like that without your own personal chef is close to impossible.

Even so, you need enough variety that your taste buds will be satisfied, but not so much that you can't sustain the time and effort that goes into making a lot of different meals. Plus, you need to keep it manageable enough that you'll be able to prep and cook your meals in bulk or ahead of time.

What I've found is that most people have the same one to three breakfasts, one to three lunches, and up to seven different dinners each week. Of course, they might change all this up if they're tired of certain foods and dishes.

When it comes to some meals, especially breakfast, I'm pretty boring! I usually eat my slow-cooker oatmeal (see page 149), egg whites, and berries every single morning. But this routine is what I need for my busy days. It's yummy, too, and makes me feel so good.

Everyone is different with regard to variety, but the Power Plate Diet gives you the ability to create daily meals that suit your preferences.

Gather Power Plate Recipes You Love

Power Plates includes lots of healthy recipes that taste amazing. I encourage you to try as many as possible and develop some favorites that you like to eat week after week.

Find at least enough recipes or simple combo ideas (examples: eggs, oatmeal, and fruit for breakfast, pasta salads or sandwiches for lunch, Slow-Cooker Beef with Broccoli (page 175) for dinner) to account for your major meals of the day. Successful meal planning comes from choosing recipes that you and your family love. Weekly favorites at my house are Cauliflower Crust BBQ Pizza (page 183) and Lettuce Wrap Street Tacos (page 186), so we go for these like crazy.

Embrace Leftovers

Many of my recipes make multiple servings, so you're bound to have leftovers. Account for eating your leftovers to minimize food waste. You can also intentionally make a double recipe for a meal, knowing you'll use the leftovers later. This makes planning, prepping, and cooking a little easier. If you have little to no time to cook for lunch, this is a great meal to schedule in leftovers. Likewise, if dinner is the meal that you have the least time to cook and prep, plan the easiest meal (or leftovers) for the dinner hour.

Get creative, too. I love omelets, for example, with all different kinds of veggies. They are quick, easy, filling, and super-clean energy for my body. I cook them in a nonstick pan with three egg whites and one whole egg—and add leftover veggies for the filling.

You can do so much with leftovers! Last night's protein can make a great base for tonight's lettuce tacos or as a topping for a lunch salad. Leftovers can make an otherwise ordinary or repetitive meal extraordinary.

Treats and Snacks

Power Plates has lots of recipes for treats and snacks. You can enjoy them between meals, and some make terrific desserts. But don't have treats containing starchy carbs at dinner—save those for earlier in the day. Using snacks between your main meals is a great way to pump up your nutrient quota and stay well-fueled for workouts.

My Beet Juice Booster

I don't go a single day without my beet juice (see page 194). It really gives me a shot of energy without the jitters. I suggest that you drink this twice a day, every day, with food, for energy and anti-inflammatory nutrition. This juice can be taken in addition to your two daily snacks, or to replace them. Add collagen peptides to your shots, too.

Plant-Based Options

Are you a vegan or vegetarian? Or are you looking for ways to incorporate more plant-based meals in your week? Power Plates has you covered! Lots of my recipes are plant-based, and are marked as VF in the recipe chapter. This makes it easy to plan your meals around your vegan or vegetarian lifestyle.

With the following sample four-week meal plan, get ready to fat-proof your body, drop inches and pounds, feel more energetic, and enjoy your food like never before. Remember, you can follow this plan to the letter, or modify it using my Power Plate guidelines. Just make sure your meals and snacks are Power Plate–approved!

WEEK ONE

Day 1

BREAKFAST: Avocado Toast on Ezekiel Bread with Eggs
(page 137)

LUNCH: Grilled chicken atop salad greens, drizzled with olive oil
and a little vinegar, and a medium baked potato

DINNER: Honey Sesame Seared Salmon with Spicy Cabbage Slaw
(page 169)

SNACK 1: 3 Peanut Butter Energy Balls (page 191)

SNACK 2: Raw power veggies and 2 tablespoons of hummus

Day 2

BREAKFAST: Egg white omelet with chopped spinach, diced
tomatoes, and chopped onions and a slice of whole-grain toast

LUNCH: Buddha bowl filled one-third with legumes or tofu, one-
third with rice, and one-third with non-starchy veggies

DINNER: Leftover Honey Sesame Seared Salmon with Spicy Cabbage Slaw (page 169)

SNACK 1: 3 Peanut Butter Energy Balls (page 191)

SNACK 2: 1 serving of air-popped popcorn

Day 3

BREAKFAST: Quinoa Porridge (page 138)

LUNCH: Tuna Salad Sandwich (page 164)

DINNER: Slow-Cooker Beef with Broccoli (page 175)

SNACK 1: A piece of fresh fruit and handful of almonds

SNACK 2: Beets and Tart Cherry Smoothie (page 195)

Day 4

BREAKFAST: Small carton of almond yogurt, oatmeal, and sliced berries

LUNCH: Healthy Egg Salad Wrap (page 165)

DINNER: Leftover Slow-Cooker Beef with Broccoli (page 175)

SNACK 1: 1 Protein Berry Muffin (page 197)

SNACK 2: Sliced apple with almond butter

Day 5

BREAKFAST: Southwestern Breakfast Burrito (page 143)

LUNCH: Creamy Avocado Chicken Salad Wrap (page 160)

DINNER: Small sirloin steak, roasted asparagus, and mashed cauliflower (microwaved from frozen package)

SNACK 1: 1 Black Bean Brownie (page 192)

SNACK 2: A piece of fresh fruit

Day 6

BREAKFAST: Scrambled eggs, a slice of rye toast, and a half grapefruit

LUNCH: A sandwich wrap filled with grilled chicken or tuna, sprouts, and sliced avocado

DINNER: Turkey Meatballs with Zucchini Noodles and Avocado Sauce (page 173), or if you want to go meatless at dinner: Szechuan Eggplant (page 188)

SNACK 1: A piece of fresh fruit

SNACK 2: 1 Black Bean Brownie (page 192)

Day 7

BREAKFAST: Sweet Plantain Waffles (page 139)

LUNCH: Spicy Lentil and Sweet Potato Salad with Vinaigrette (page 151)

DINNER: Pesto Whitefish Packet with Veggies (page 176)

SNACK 1: Raw power veggies and 2 tablespoons of hummus

SNACK 2: Pumpkin Protein Smoothie (page 197)

WEEK TWO

Day 8

BREAKFAST: Smoked salmon, a whole-grain English muffin, a slice of red onion, and capers

LUNCH: Beet and Bean Burger (page 166)

DINNER: Leftover Pesto Whitefish Packet with Veggies (page 176)

SNACK 1: 2 hard-boiled eggs

SNACK 2: 1 Pumpkin Bar (page 200)

Day 9

BREAKFAST: Chia Seed Pudding (page 138)

LUNCH: Quinoa Pasta with Pan-Seared Chicken and Creamy Avocado Spinach Sauce (page 152)

DINNER: Grilled chicken breast, one-half baked acorn squash, and spinach sautéed in a little olive oil

SNACK 1: 2 hard-boiled eggs

SNACK 2: 1 Pumpkin Bar (page 200)

Day 10

BREAKFAST: Scrambled egg whites, quinoa, and a half grapefruit

LUNCH: Barley Salad with Lemony Kale Pesto (page 156)

DINNER: Cauliflower Crust BBQ Pizza (page 183)

SNACK 1: 1 serving of Healthy Freezer Fudge (page 198)

SNACK 2: A piece of fresh fruit and handful of walnuts

Day 11

BREAKFAST: Egg Muffin with Whole-Grain Toast (page 144)

LUNCH: Lean ground beef patty on a whole-grain bun with a sliced tomato

DINNER: Chicken Alfredo Spaghetti Squash (page 179), or if you want to go meatless: Quick and Easy Black Bean Enchiladas (page 189)

SNACK 1: 1 serving of Healthy Freezer Fudge (page 198)

SNACK 2: 6-ounce carton of almond milk yogurt over a sliced banana

Day 12

BREAKFAST: Scrambled egg whites, a slice of Ezekiel bread toast, and a bowl of mixed berries

LUNCH: Roasted chicken breast, roasted asparagus, and a baked potato

DINNER: Crunchy Coconut and Kale Salmon (page 180)

SNACK 1: 1 serving of air-popped popcorn

SNACK 2: 1 or 2 Banana Oatmeal Cookies (page 199)

Day 13

BREAKFAST: Power Oats (page 141)

LUNCH: Quinoa-Stuffed Acorn Squash (page 163)

DINNER: Lean ground beef cooked in unsweetened pasta sauce and served atop steamed spiralized zucchini (for convenience, use the microwavable spirals from the frozen foods section)

SNACK 1: Handful of toasted almonds

SNACK 2: 1 or 2 Banana Oatmeal Cookies (page 199)

Day 14

BREAKFAST: Almond Flour Pancakes (page 141)

LUNCH: ¾ cup hummus and sliced cucumbers and quartered whole-grain pita bread for dipping

DINNER: Curry Chicken Lettuce Wrap (page 171)

SNACK 1: Handful of Tart Cherry Lime Gummies (page 202)

SNACK 2: Apple slices with almond butter

Day 15

BREAKFAST: Smoked salmon, whole-grain bagel, slice of red onion, and capers

LUNCH: Savory Steel-Cut Oats with Fried Egg (page 153)

DINNER: Steak Salad with Rosemary Olive Oil Dressing (page 185)

SNACK 1: Any of my smoothies (see pages 195–97)

SNACK 2: 1 slice Healthy Banana Nut Bread (page 193)

Day 16

BREAKFAST: Mashed Banana Oatmeal (page 140)

LUNCH: Grilled shrimp atop salad greens, drizzled with olive oil and a little vinegar, and a side of quinoa

DINNER: Low-Carb Chicken Pad Thai with Vegetable Noodles (page 177)

SNACK 1: Handful of toasted almonds

SNACK 2: 1 slice Healthy Banana Nut Bread (page 193)

Day 17

BREAKFAST: Scrambled egg whites and oatmeal topped with fresh berries

LUNCH: Roasted Butternut Squash Pecan Quinoa Salad (page 154)

DINNER: Leftover Low-Carb Chicken Pad Thai with Vegetable Noodles (page 177)

SNACK 1: Creamy Avocado and Mint Smoothie (page 196)

SNACK 2: A piece of fresh fruit

Day 18

BREAKFAST: Overnight Steel-Cut Oats (page 149)

LUNCH: Buddha bowl filled one-third with legumes or tofu, one-third with rice, and one-third with low-starch veggies

DINNER: Chicken Zoodle Soup (page 182)

SNACK 1: 1 serving of Banana Ice Cream (page 194)

SNACK 2: A piece of fresh fruit

Day 19

BREAKFAST: Egg white omelet with chopped spinach, diced tomatoes, and chopped onions and a slice of whole-grain toast

LUNCH: Leftover Chicken Zoodle Soup (page 182) and a slice of whole-grain bread or a medium baked potato

DINNER: Salmon and Scallops Salad (page 187), or if you want to go meatless: Stuffed Poblano Peppers (page 190)

SNACK 1: 1 serving of Banana Ice Cream (page 194)

SNACK 2: Handful of toasted nuts

Day 20

BREAKFAST: Banana Cinnamon Pancakes (page 145)

LUNCH: Quinoa, Tempeh, and Roasted Veggie Salad with Walnut Dressing (page 157)

DINNER: Restaurant meal—Power Plate–approved

SNACK 1: Handful of toasted nuts

SNACK 2: 1 slice of Dessert Pizza (page 200)

Day 21

BREAKFAST: Turkey sausage, a slice of whole-grain toast, and fresh berries

LUNCH: Leftover Quinoa, Tempeh, and Roasted Veggie Salad with Walnut Dressing (page 157)

DINNER: Chicken Enchilada Cauliflower Rice Bowl (page 172)

SNACK 1: Raw power veggies and 2 tablespoons of hummus

SNACK 2: 1 slice of Dessert Pizza (page 200)

WEEK FOUR

Day 22

BREAKFAST: Acai Breakfast Bowl (page 150)

LUNCH: Lentil Pasta with Butternut Squash "Cheesy" Sauce (page 155)

DINNER: Grilled salmon or other seafood, mashed parsnips, and roasted Brussels sprouts

SNACK 1: Raw power veggies and 2 tablespoons of hummus

SNACK 2: 6-ounce carton of almond milk yogurt

Day 23

BREAKFAST: Turkey sausage, a slice of whole-grain toast, and fresh berries

LUNCH: Leftover Lentil Pasta with Butternut Squash "Cheesy" Sauce (page 155)

DINNER: Lettuce Wrap Street Tacos (page 186)

SNACK 1: ½ cup of steamed edamame

SNACK 2: A piece of fresh fruit and handful of almonds or walnuts

Day 24

BREAKFAST: Breakfast Quiche with Sweet Potato Crust (page 146)

LUNCH: Strawberry Spinach Salad with Tofu and Simple Dressing (page 158)

DINNER: Leftover Lettuce Wrap Street Tacos (page 186)

SNACK 1: 2 No-Bake Cheesecake Bites (page 201)

SNACK 2: ½ cup steamed edamame

Day 25

BREAKFAST: Leftover Breakfast Quiche with Sweet Potato Crust (page 146)

LUNCH: Quinoa-Stuffed Acorn Squash (page 163)

DINNER: Stir-fried vegetables with cauliflower rice and tofu or edamame

SNACK 1: 2 No-Bake Cheesecake Bites (page 201)

SNACK 2: A piece of fresh fruit and handful of almonds or walnuts

Day 26

BREAKFAST: Pan-fried turkey sausage and oatmeal topped with blueberries

LUNCH: Shredded Brussels Sprouts and Kale Salad with Roasted Sweet Potatoes and Almond Butter Dressing (page 162)

DINNER: Cauli-Fried Rice with Eggs and Veggies (page 184)

SNACK 1: 3 Peanut Butter Energy Balls (page 191)

SNACK 2: Any of my smoothies (see pages 195–97)

Day 27

BREAKFAST: Breakfast Casserole with Sweet Potatoes, Broccoli, and Peppers (page 148)

LUNCH: Leftover Shredded Brussels Sprouts and Kale Salad with Roasted Sweet Potatoes and Almond Butter (page 162)

DINNER: Restaurant meal—Power Plate–approved

SNACK 1: 3 Peanut Butter Energy Balls (page 191)

SNACK 2: 1 serving of air-popped popcorn

Day 28

BREAKFAST: Roasted Acorn Squash with Yogurt, Honey, and Nuts (page 147)

LUNCH: Broiled Orange Teriyaki Salmon with Edamame and Quinoa (page 161)

DINNER: Leftover Cauli-Fried Rice with Eggs and Veggies (page 184)

SNACK 1: Apple slices with almond or peanut butter

SNACK 2: Any of my smoothies (see pages 195–97)

Stress-Free Grocery Shopping

Does grocery shopping overwhelm you? Is it hard to find time for trips to the store? Or are you always making runs to the grocery store for items you forgot?

Shopping for groceries doesn't have to be time-consuming or stressful if you're well-prepared. Like you, I'm super-busy, but I've found ways to streamline my shopping so that I have plenty of time for my family, fun activities, and everything else going on in my life.

For starters, the simplest way to grocery shop is to use my app, Pretty Muscles. It can load up a grocery cart with the ingredients you need and then ship those directly to you. It's so simple, and you can find my great Power Plate–approved recipes on there, too.

In addition, here's what I've learned (mostly through trial and error!) that has helped me over the years.

SHOP MOSTLY AT THE SAME STORE. This is a biggie! If you've ever shopped for groceries in an unfamiliar store, you know the frustration. Where the heck are the spices, the beans, the condiments? You spend more time looking for stuff than actually selecting it. I used to be like that, and I'd always find myself wandering aimlessly around the store.

Then I got smart. Now I'm familiar with the grocery store that I shop at. Consequently, I go from one part of the grocery store straight to another until everything on my list is in my grocery cart. So stick with your favorite store. You'll be in and out in no time.

STAY MOSTLY ON THE PERIMETER OF THE STORE. The healthiest foods—like vegetables, fruits, and lean proteins—are on the outer aisles of the store. Spend most of your time there and less time in the center aisles where junk foods and processed foods lurk.

STOCK UP ON STAPLES. Check the grocery shelves for Power Plate–approved nonperishables you can store in your pantry and freezer: canned and bottled goods; dried beans and legumes; frozen vegetables and fruits; approved pastas, quinoa, oats, and brown rice; nuts and nut butters, and so forth.

DON'T SHOP ON AN EMPTY STOMACH. Grocery shopping when I'm hungry never ends well for me or my bank account. I find it hard to concentrate when famished. All I can think about is getting something to eat, and the impulse buying begins. It's like going sight-seeing in the tropics and suddenly having to pee—finding a restroom becomes more important than the incredible views. As I put away my groceries at home, I end up wondering "What was I thinking?" Lesson: Have a meal or snack before going to the grocery store.

WORK FROM A SHOPPING LIST. Plan your weekly menus in advance, and build a shopping list from those. You can adapt the shopping list I've created (see opposite page); I generated it from my suggested meal plans. It allows you to check off items you need to purchase and write in the quantity.

We use a family app called Cozi, too, which allows everyone in the family to add to our grocery list. When I'm at the store, I just pull up the list, and I see what we need.

The Power Plates Shopping List

The shopping lists that follow cover all four weeks' worth of sample menus. How many ingredients you'll actually purchase depends on how many people you're cooking for. So generally, if you're cooking for one or two, you'd buy much less than if you're preparing meals for an entire family.

Some of my recipes call for multiple servings, which will feed a family or you can save the extra servings for another meal or two. (See my meal prep suggestions on page 131.) If you want a single serving, simply cut the recipe down. The number of servings each recipe yields is located in the recipe, so you're never in doubt about how many servings the listed ingredients will provide. Thus, the amounts are just a baseline from which you can multiply and reduce as you need.

Also, whether you cook just a few of the recipes or a lot of them will determine the foods you buy and the quantities. It's best to review the meal plans, decide on which meals you'll prepare and which recipes you'll use, then check off what you need using this list.

If you bought everything on the list, you'd end up with more food than you need—which is why I recommend planning your meals. And if you find that you have more than enough, freeze extra meats, vegetables, fruits, and leftovers, and you'll save time and money.

The list is set up so that you can check off what you need and fill in the amounts.

POWER PROTEINS

☐ Beans and legumes, such as black beans, canned _____

☐ Beef, sirloin or other lean cuts _____

☐ Chicken breasts, boneless, skinless _____

☐ Chicken, shredded _____

☐ Chicken or turkey sausage _____

- [ ] Edamame _____
- [ ] Eggs _____
- [ ] Hummus _____
- [ ] Lentils _____
- [ ] Mussels _____
- [ ] Other meats (bison, pork, or lamb) _____
- [ ] Oysters _____
- [ ] Salmon, smoked _____
- [ ] Salmon, wild-caught _____
- [ ] Sardines _____
- [ ] Scallops, fresh or frozen _____
- [ ] Shrimp _____
- [ ] Tempeh _____
- [ ] Tofu _____
- [ ] Tuna, wild-caught, canned _____
- [ ] Turkey, ground, lean _____
- [ ] Whitefish, any type _____

POWER CARBS

- [ ] Breads
  - [ ] Brown rice wraps _____
  - [ ] Cauliflower flatbreads or tortillas _____
  - [ ] Sprouted-grain bread (Ezekiel) _____
  - [ ] Whole-grain or whole-wheat bread _____
  - [ ] Whole-grain or whole-wheat hamburger buns _____
  - [ ] Whole-wheat pita bread _____
  - [ ] Whole-wheat tortillas and wraps _____

- [ ] Grains
  - [ ] Amaranth _____
  - [ ] Barley _____
  - [ ] Brown rice _____
  - [ ] Buckwheat _____
  - [ ] Bulgur _____
  - [ ] Cassava _____
  - [ ] Farro _____
  - [ ] Granola, low sugar _____
  - [ ] Kamut wheat _____
  - [ ] Millet _____
  - [ ] Oats, old-fashioned and steel cut _____
  - [ ] Quinoa _____
  - [ ] Wheat berries _____
- [ ] Pastas
  - [ ] Lentil pasta _____
  - [ ] Quinoa pasta _____
  - [ ] Whole-wheat pasta _____
- [ ] Starchy and low-starch starchy vegetables
  - [ ] Acorn squash _____
  - [ ] Butternut squash _____
  - [ ] Corn _____
  - [ ] Parsnips _____
  - [ ] Peas _____
  - [ ] Popcorn (stovetop) _____
  - [ ] Potatoes _____
  - [ ] Pumpkin puree, canned _____

- [ ] Spaghetti squash _____
- [ ] Sweet potatoes or yams _____

POWER PRODUCE—NON-STARCHY VEGETABLES

- [ ] Arugula _____
- [ ] Beets _____
- [ ] Belgian endive _____
- [ ] Bell pepper, any color _____
- [ ] Bok choy _____
- [ ] Broccoli _____
- [ ] Brussels sprouts _____
- [ ] Cabbage, green and red _____
- [ ] Carrots _____
- [ ] Cauliflower, fresh _____
- [ ] Cauliflower rice, frozen _____
- [ ] Celery _____
- [ ] Collards _____
- [ ] Cucumbers _____
- [ ] Eggplant _____
- [ ] Garlic _____
- [ ] Green chilies, canned _____
- [ ] Jalapeño peppers _____
- [ ] Jicama _____
- [ ] Kale _____
- [ ] Kale, lacinato _____
- [ ] Kelp _____
- [ ] Leeks _____

☐ Lettuce, any type including butter, Bibb, and romaine _____

☐ Mixed vegetables, stir-fry, frozen _____

☐ Mushrooms, shiitake, portobello, button _____

☐ Onions, green _____

☐ Onions, red and white _____

☐ Poblano peppers _____

☐ Radicchio leaves _____

☐ Radishes _____

☐ Scallions _____

☐ Shallots _____

☐ Spinach _____

☐ Spinach, baby _____

☐ Spring greens _____

☐ Sprouts, any type _____

☐ Swiss chard _____

☐ Tomatoes _____

☐ Tomatoes, cherry _____

☐ Water chestnuts _____

☐ Zucchini _____

☐ Other low-starch, high-fiber vegetables _____

POWER PRODUCE—FRUITS

☐ Acai berries _____

☐ Acai puree _____

☐ Apples _____

☐ Apples, green _____

☐ Applesauce, unsweetened _____

☐ Apricots _____

☐ Avocados _____

☐ Bananas _____

☐ Blueberries _____

☐ Cantaloupe _____

☐ Cherries, pitted, frozen, unsweetened _____

☐ Cranberries _____

☐ Currants _____

☐ Dates _____

☐ Figs _____

☐ Grapefruit _____

☐ Grapes _____

☐ Guava _____

☐ Kiwi _____

☐ Lemons _____

☐ Limes _____

☐ Mangoes _____

☐ Oranges _____

☐ Papaya _____

☐ Peaches _____

☐ Pineapple _____

☐ Plantains _____

☐ Plums _____

☐ Prunes _____

☐ Raisins _____

☐ Raspberries _____

- [ ] Strawberries _____
- [ ] Tart cherry juice _____
- [ ] Watermelon _____

POWER FATS

- [ ] Almond butter _____
- [ ] Avocado oil _____
- [ ] Coconut oil, liquid _____
- [ ] Coconut oil, solid _____
- [ ] Grapeseed oil _____
- [ ] Macadamia nut oil _____
- [ ] Olive oil, preferably extra-virgin _____
- [ ] Peanut butter, natural _____
- [ ] Safflower oil _____
- [ ] Sesame oil _____
- [ ] Sunflower oil _____
- [ ] Vegenaise _____
- [ ] Vegetable oil cooking spray _____

NUTS AND SEEDS

- [ ] Almonds, sliced or whole _____
- [ ] Cashews, raw _____
- [ ] Chia seeds _____
- [ ] Coconut, shredded, unsweetened _____
- [ ] Flaxseeds _____
- [ ] Hazelnuts _____

- ☐ Hemp seeds _____
- ☐ Peanuts _____
- ☐ Pecans, halved _____
- ☐ Pine nuts _____
- ☐ Pistachios _____
- ☐ Pumpkin seeds (pepitas), hulled _____
- ☐ Sesame seeds _____
- ☐ Sunflower seeds _____
- ☐ Walnuts _____

FRESH HERBS

- ☐ Basil _____
- ☐ Chives _____
- ☐ Cilantro _____
- ☐ Dill _____
- ☐ Ginger _____
- ☐ Mint _____
- ☐ Parsley _____
- ☐ Rosemary _____
- ☐ Thyme _____

DRIED HERBS AND SPICES

In addition to the spices listed on page 86, the following are used in my recipes.

- ☐ Black pepper _____
- ☐ Cayenne pepper _____
- ☐ Chili powder _____

- [ ] Cinnamon, ground _____
- [ ] Coriander, ground _____
- [ ] Cumin, ground _____
- [ ] Garlic powder _____
- [ ] Ginger, ground _____
- [ ] Onion powder _____
- [ ] Paprika, smoked _____
- [ ] Pumpkin pie spice _____
- [ ] Red pepper flakes _____
- [ ] Rosemary, dried _____
- [ ] Salt _____
- [ ] Thyme, dried _____
- [ ] Turmeric, ground _____

NON-DAIRY FOODS

- [ ] Almond milk, unsweetened _____
- [ ] Almond milk yogurt _____
- [ ] Coconut milk, unsweetened _____

CONDIMENTS, VINEGARS, AND FLAVORING

- [ ] Adobe sauce _____
- [ ] Coconut aminos _____
- [ ] Enchilada sauce, green, low-sodium _____
- [ ] Enchilada sauce, red, low-sodium _____
- [ ] Fish sauce _____
- [ ] Green Goddess salad dressing, low sugar, low sodium _____
- [ ] Hot sauce _____

- [ ] Mustards:
  - [ ] Brown _____
  - [ ] Dijon _____
  - [ ] Regular _____
  - [ ] Spicy _____
- [ ] Pasta sauce, unsweetened _____
- [ ] Szechuan sauce, spicy _____
- [ ] Tomato puree _____
- [ ] Vanilla extract _____
- [ ] Vinegars:
  - [ ] Apple cider _____
  - [ ] Balsamic _____
  - [ ] Red wine _____
  - [ ] Rice wine _____
  - [ ] White wine _____

SWEETENERS

- [ ] Agave nectar _____
- [ ] Coconut nectar _____
- [ ] Coconut sugar _____
- [ ] Honey _____
- [ ] Maple syrup _____
- [ ] Stevia _____
- [ ] Swerve _____
- [ ] Truvia _____

FLOURS

- [ ] Almond flour _____
- [ ] Coconut flour _____

SUPPLEMENTS

- [ ] Collagen peptides _____

OTHER

- [ ] Arrowroot or tapioca _____
- [ ] Baking powder _____
- [ ] Baking soda _____
- [ ] Black olives _____
- [ ] Broth (chicken), low-sodium _____
- [ ] Cacao nibs _____
- [ ] Cocoa powder, unsweetened _____
- [ ] Dark chocolate chips _____
- [ ] Gelatin powder _____
- [ ] Greek yogurt _____
- [ ] Mozzarella cheese _____
- [ ] Nutritional yeast _____
- [ ] Pre-made cauliflower crusts _____
- [ ] Pre-made cauliflower thins _____
- [ ] Vegan cream cheese _____

Prep Day!

Want to save precious time during the week? Schedule a "Prep Day" when you get most of your food ready to go for the week ahead.

My husband and I have been doing Prep Days for years, so we have it down to a science. Certain foods are worth the time and energy it takes to prep them for the week. Other foods aren't worth it, especially those that come pre-sliced, pre-cut, or pre-cooked already. Sure, you're paying for convenience, but you salvage a lot of extra time.

Our Prep Day is usually Sunday. Your own Prep Day is up to you and should fit your daily routine. With a weekly Prep Day, you not only save time, but you also automatically fix more nutritious meal choices for the long term.

There are different ways to meal prep, and I use a combination of all of these:

MAKE-AHEAD MEALS: Prepare some full meals for the week ahead—meals that can be refrigerated and reheated. This type of prep comes in handy for dinners.

BATCH COOKING: You can also cook up large batches of recipes, split them into individual portions to be frozen, and eat them over the next few months.

READY-TO-COOK INGREDIENTS: This is my most-used strategy. I prep the ingredients required for specific meals ahead of time in order to cut down on my cooking time.

My Prep Day involves the following foods:

EGGS. If I'm not scrambling them or making omelets, I'm hard-boiling them for snacks or to use on salads. Or I just buy them already hard-boiled!

GRAINS. Many grains, including rice, quinoa, and oats, can be cooked ahead of time. I then store them in the refrigerator or freezer for quick reheating throughout the week.

PEPPERS. I love to dice up raw peppers and refrigerate them in an airtight container. I toss them into omelets, salads, tacos, and on top of cauliflower pizza.

NUTS. I'm a fan of toasted nuts for salad toppings, veggie dish toppings, and grab-and-go snacking. Place your almonds, pecans, walnuts, pine nuts, and others in individual rows on a cookie sheet and bake them at 425ºF for 8 to 10 minutes.

GRAPES. These babies go bad fast in the fridge, so I like to freeze them and eat them as a sweet frozen snack. If you don't like them frozen, just pull them off the vine and place them in a plastic container. Super-quick and easy snack when you don't have to pluck!

BANANAS. Likewise, bananas turn brown and mushy fast. Solution: Wrap them in aluminum foil or peel them and place them in a zip-top plastic storage bag, then pop them in the freezer. Use them frozen, or in my Banana Ice Cream. Never toss out a banana again!

BERRIES. After washing them, put them into a clear airtight container. They'll last longer. Or you can freeze them. Either way, use them in smoothies, on cereal, and in salads.

LETTUCE. Keep lettuce and other greens like spinach fresh in their containers by placing a paper towel over the leaves and closing the container. This trick is a miracle move—no more wilted, ugly greens. Alternatively, chop up lettuces like romaine and bag them yourself. (You'll want to keep some lettuces intact, though, for lettuce leaf wraps.)

BEETS. Roast this superfood ahead of time so you can use them throughout the week as salad toppings, in vegetable wraps, or as an earthy side dish at lunch or dinner. But if you're going to make beet juice, keep them fresh. Don't cook them.

CHICKEN. Cook at least part of your weekly supply of chicken, whether you like to grill, bake, or roast it. I love to sear mine with good heat from red pepper flakes on an electric skillet. Picking up a rotisserie chicken at the grocery store is a super time-saver. I can tear off pieces—sans skin—for salads, wraps, and stir-fries. I'll bring the rotisserie chicken home and immediately pull the meat off and place it in a container for easy grabbing later.

EGG CASSEROLE. I like to make a large casserole pan of eggs, sautéed veggies, ground turkey sausage, and a little crispy bacon. Then I cut it into grabbable squares and store it in the fridge for easy and tasty munching!

MUFFINS AND OTHER TREATS. Many of my snacks can be stored in the fridge or frozen for an anytime-mini-meal or to grab as you fly out the door like I do.

Happy Prep Day!

7

THE POWER PLATE DIET RECIPES

Part of the beauty of Power Plates is that they give you meals and recipes that are so delicious that you won't even realize you're trying to slim down. Why sit down to a plain chicken breast and soggy veggies when you can be digging in to a juicy lean steak or crispy seared chicken tenders with subtly sweet, tasty squash, a fresh bed of greens, and a yummy dessert? If you're bored with your food, you're eating the wrong food. So say goodbye to bland, boring meals with these recipes.

Note: The VF designation means that the recipe is vegan- or vegetarian-friendly and appropriate for a plant-based meal or menu.

POWER PLATE KITCHEN TOOLS

Besides your basic kitchen tools like saucepans and skillets, it helps to have the following on hand, too:

Baking sheets and pans

Food processor

Grater

Griddle

High-speed blender

Juicer

Large electric skillet

Mandoline

Outdoor electric grill

Parchment paper

Slow cooker

Spiralizer or vegetable peeler

Waffle maker

Whisks

COOKING SWAPS I LOVE

All-purpose white flour	100% whole-wheat flour, almond flour, coconut flour, whole-grain oat flour, or spelt flour
Butter or margarine in baked goods	Coconut oil, ♥unsweetened applesauce, or mashed or pureed avocado. (These work in a 1:1 ratio—a half cup for a half cup of butter.)
Sugar in baked goods*	♥Maple syrup, honey, agave nectar, and the zero-calorie sweeteners stevia, ♥Truvia, or Swerve

♥These items are my favorites and are always in my fridge and pantry.

*****NOTE:** When substituting maple syrup in baked goods, use about ⅔ cup to ¾ cup syrup per cup of sugar. With agave nectar, use one-third less than you would sugar and reduce other liquids in the recipe by one-quarter. With honey, use about ⅔ cup to ¾ cup per cup of sugar. As for the zero-calorie sweeteners, see the package directions for how to replace sugar in recipes.

Avocado Toast on Ezekiel Bread
with Eggs

SERVES: 1
TIME: 5 minutes

Vegetable oil cooking spray
1 whole egg + 2 egg whites
½ avocado, peeled and pitted
1 teaspoon freshly squeezed lemon juice
⅛ teaspoon salt
Black pepper
1 slice Ezekiel bread, toasted

In a skillet that has been lightly coated with vegetable oil cooking spray, fry the egg and egg whites over medium heat. Scoop out the avocado flesh and mash it in a bowl with the lemon juice, salt, and black pepper to taste. Spread the avocado mixture on the toasted Ezekiel bread and top with the eggs to serve.

Quinoa Porridge

SERVES: 2
TIME: 20 minutes

1 cup quinoa, rinsed and strained

1 apple, peeled and diced

1½ cups unsweetened almond milk

1 teaspoon ground cinnamon

½ teaspoon vanilla extract

2 tablespoons maple syrup

¼ cup coarsely chopped walnuts (optional)

4 egg whites, scrambled

Add the quinoa to a medium-sized pot, along with half of the diced apple, the almond milk, ½ cup of water, and the cinnamon. Bring to a boil over high heat, then reduce to medium heat to simmer until almost all the liquid is absorbed, 10 to 15 minutes. Remove from the heat and stir in the vanilla extract and maple syrup. Top with the remaining apples and walnuts (if using). Serve alongside the scrambled egg whites.

Chia Seed Pudding

VF

SERVES: 2

TIME: 10 minutes, plus at least 2 hours in the refrigerator

6 tablespoons chia seeds

½ cup old-fashioned oats

2 cups unsweetened almond or coconut milk

½ teaspoon vanilla extract

1 tablespoon honey (or maple syrup or coconut nectar if vegan)

Small handful blueberries or raspberries

In a bowl, mix together the chia seeds, oats, almond or coconut milk, vanilla extract, and honey until well combined. Divide between two serving bowls or mason jars, and place in the refrigerator to set for at least 2 hours or overnight. Once the pudding has a thick consistency, top with berries and serve.

Sweet Plantain Waffles

VF

SERVES: 2

TIME: 15 minutes

2 cups mashed ripe plantains

2½ tablespoons coconut oil, melted

1 teaspoon ground cinnamon

1 teaspoon vanilla extract

1 teaspoon apple cider vinegar

½ teaspoon baking soda

Vegetable oil cooking spray (optional)

TOPPINGS (OPTIONAL)

Almond butter

Maple syrup

Fresh berries

Preheat a waffle maker to high heat. Add the plantains to a high-speed blender or food processor and blend until smooth. Add in the melted coconut oil, cinnamon, vanilla, and apple cider vinegar, then pulse until smooth and incorporated. Add the baking soda and mix again until incorporated.

Lightly oil the waffle maker with vegetable oil cooking spray or oil if needed, and pour ⅓ cup batter onto the heated griddle. Let cook for 2 to 3 minutes until desired doneness, and repeat with the remaining batter. (You may need to grease the waffle maker in between batches.) Let the waffles cool slightly on a wire rack before serving. To serve, top with almond butter for extra protein as well as maple syrup and fresh berries, if desired.

Mashed Banana Oatmeal

VF

SERVES: 2

TIME: 15 minutes

1 cup unsweetened almond milk
⅓ cup mashed banana
⅛ teaspoon ground cinnamon
2 cups barley
1 tablespoon old-fashioned oats
1 tablespoon collagen peptides (omit if vegan)
Fresh berries

In a medium pot, whisk together the almond milk, mashed banana, and cinnamon. Cook over medium heat, stirring, until thickened slightly. Add the frozen barley and the oats and continue cooking until the grains are heated through and the porridge is thickened.

Remove from the heat and stir in the collagen peptides. Divide into serving bowls and top with fresh berries to serve.

Power Oats

VF

SERVES: 2

TIME: 10 minutes

1 cup old-fashioned oats

2 tablespoons collagen peptides (omit if vegan)

1 banana, sliced

2 tablespoons natural peanut butter

2 tablespoons hemp seeds

½ cup strawberries, sliced

In a medium pot, bring 2 cups of water to a boil over high heat. Add in the oats and reduce heat to medium to let simmer for 5 minutes, or until most of the water is absorbed. Stir in the collagen peptides, then divide between two serving bowls.

Top both servings with the banana slices, peanut butter, hemp seeds, and sliced strawberries. Serve immediately, eating either as is or stirring everything together.

Almond Flour Pancakes

SERVES: 2 to 4

TIME: 15 minutes

1½ cups almond flour

½ cup tapioca starch or arrowroot starch

½ teaspoon ground cinnamon

¾ cup unsweetened almond milk

3 eggs

1 teaspoon honey (or maple syrup or coconut nectar if vegan)

Vegetable oil cooking spray

TOPPINGS (OPTIONAL)

Plain Greek yogurt

Blueberries

Sliced banana

Chia seeds

In a large mixing bowl, whisk together the almond flour, tapioca starch, and cinnamon.

In a separate, smaller bowl, whisk together the almond milk, eggs, and honey. Add the egg mixture to the almond flour mixture and whisk everything together until no clumps remain.

Heat a griddle or skillet over medium heat with cooking spray or a little oil. Use a measuring cup to scoop ¼ cup batter onto the griddle. Cook for 2 to 3 minutes on one side. Flip and cook for another 2 minutes. Repeat with the remaining batter. Serve immediately and top with yogurt, blueberries, banana, and chia seeds, as desired.

> TIP: Curious about the use of tapioca and arrowroot starches? This is what will bind the pancakes together as well as provide the starch component for earlier in the day. They are also a source of resistant starch, which contributes to good gut health.

Southwestern Breakfast Burrito

SERVES: 4

TIME: 20 minutes

Vegetable oil cooking spray (optional)

4 (8-inch) whole-wheat tortillas

1 (15-ounce) can black beans, rinsed and drained

4 eggs, scrambled

⅛ teaspoon black pepper

½ red onion, diced

¼ cup chopped fresh cilantro (optional)

½ cup plain Greek yogurt

Preheat the oven to 400°F.

Place parchment paper on a baking sheet or lightly oil the baking sheet with cooking spray and set aside.

Lay out the whole-wheat tortillas and layer with the black beans, scrambled eggs, pepper, diced onion, and chopped cilantro (if using). Roll up burrito-style so that both ends are sealed.

Place on the prepared baking sheet and bake for 10 to 15 minutes until heated thoroughly. Serve with plain Greek yogurt on top.

Egg Muffins with Whole-Grain Toast

SERVES: 6

TIME: 30 minutes

½ pound chicken or turkey sausage

Vegetable oil cooking spray

6 eggs

¼ cup chopped mushrooms (shiitake or button)

2 tablespoons chopped fresh basil

Ezekiel or other whole-grain toast

Preheat the oven to 350°F.

Heat a skillet over medium-high heat and sauté the sausage until cooked through and slightly golden brown, breaking it up into crumbles. Drain any excess fat and set aside.

Grease 6 cups of a standard muffin tin with vegetable oil cooking spray or oil and set aside. Crack the eggs into a large mixing bowl and whisk together. Add in the cooked sausage, mushrooms, and fresh basil, then whisk again until well incorporated. Pour even amounts of egg mixture into each muffin cup.

Bake for 20 minutes or until cooked through. Serve with your favorite whole-grain toast.

TIP: These muffins are easy to make ahead of time on your meal prep day. Then just grab the next morning for a delicious breakfast on-the-go!

Banana Cinnamon Pancakes

SERVES: 2

TIME: 10 minutes

2 bananas, plus more (optional) for topping

1 cup liquid egg whites

1 teaspoon ground cinnamon

2 tablespoons natural peanut butter or almond butter, plus more (optional) for topping

Coconut oil or vegetable oil cooking spray

1 tablespoon chia seeds

In a high-speed blender, combine the bananas, egg whites, cinnamon, and nut butter until smooth.

Heat a skillet or griddle on medium-high heat with a bit of coconut oil or cooking spray. Scoop about ⅓ cup of the batter onto the skillet and cook for 2 to 3 minutes on one side, or until bubbles form. Flip and cook for about 2 minutes, or until the pancakes are slightly brown on the edges. Remove the cooked pancake to a plate and repeat with the remaining batter.

To serve, top the pancakes with the chia seeds and additional banana slices and peanut butter, if desired.

Breakfast Quiche with Sweet Potato Crust

SERVES: 2 to 4

TIME: 35 minutes

1 sweet potato, peeled

Vegetable oil cooking spray

6 eggs

½ onion, diced

1 cup spinach

1 cup chopped mushrooms (shiitake or button)

⅛ teaspoon black pepper

½ cup unsweetened almond milk or unsweetened coconut milk

½ teaspoon garlic powder

Preheat the oven to 350ºF.

Thinly slice the sweet potato using a knife or mandoline.

Grease a quiche pan or baking dish with the cooking spray or oil and layer in the sweet potato slices, slightly overlapping each other. Whisk the eggs together in a mixing bowl and set aside.

Spray a large pan with vegetable oil cooking spray and sauté the onions, spinach, and mushrooms over medium-high heat for a few minutes until slightly cooked down. Add the sautéed vegetables to the eggs, then whisk in the black pepper, almond milk, and garlic powder.

Pour the egg mixture on top of the sliced sweet potatoes. Bake for about 30 minutes, until the eggs have set. Serve immediately.

Roasted Acorn Squash with Yogurt, Honey, and Nuts

VF

SERVES: 2

TIME: 50 minutes

1 acorn squash

1 teaspoon avocado oil

½ teaspoon ground cinnamon

1 cup plain Greek yogurt (or almond yogurt if vegan)

2 tablespoons honey (or maple syrup or coconut nectar if vegan)

¼ cup coarsely chopped walnuts

½ cup low-sugar granola (optional)

Preheat the oven to 400°F. Line a baking sheet with parchment paper.

Slice the acorn squash in half lengthwise and scoop out the seeds. Rub the avocado oil all over the skin and inside of the squash, then sprinkle with the cinnamon. Place the squash, cut side down, on the prepared baking sheet.

Bake for 40 to 45 minutes, until easily pierced with a fork. Turn the squash over and fill with the yogurt, honey, walnuts, and granola (if using). Serve.

Breakfast Casserole with Sweet Potatoes, Broccoli, and Peppers

SERVES: 4

TIME: 1 hour

Vegetable oil cooking spray

1 sweet potato, peeled and grated (about 1½ cups)

2 cups broccoli florets

1½ bell peppers, cored, seeded, and diced

6 eggs

½ cup unsweetened almond milk

Salt

½ teaspoon garlic powder

½ teaspoon onion powder

Preheat the oven to 375°F. Spray a 9 × 13-inch baking dish with vegetable oil cooking spray and set aside.

Spray a skillet and sauté the grated sweet potato, broccoli florets, and bell peppers over medium-high heat for several minutes, until slightly caramelized and browned. Remove from the heat and set aside.

In a large mixing bowl, whisk the eggs together, then add the sautéed vegetables, almond milk, salt to taste, the garlic powder, and the onion powder until well combined. Pour the egg mixture into the prepared baking dish. Bake for 45 minutes or until completely cooked through. Let sit for 10 minutes before slicing and serving.

> TIP: To save time, make this dish the night before you plan to serve it. Bake the casserole according to the instructions, then let it cool and place in the refrigerator. To reheat, put it in the oven at 350°F until heated through, 10 to 20 minutes.

Overnight Steel-Cut Oats

VF

SERVES: 4

TIME: 4 hours (you can do it overnight!)

Vegetable oil cooking spray

1 cup steel-cut oats

1 cup chopped peeled apples

½ teaspoon ground cinnamon

2 scoops collagen peptides (optional; omit if vegan)

2 teaspoons maple syrup (optional)

Lightly spray a slow cooker with vegetable oil cooking spray. Add the oats, 4 cups of water, the apples, and the cinnamon. Cook on high for 4 hours or low for 8 hours.

When you're ready to eat, scoop into four dishes and mix in ½ scoop collagen peptides and ½ teaspoon maple syrup, if using, per serving.

> TIP: They say that variety is the spice of life, but I eat this oatmeal literally every day. I prep it before I go to bed and wake up to a batch of delicious oatmeal—all it needs is a few healthy toppings!

Acai Breakfast Bowl

VF
SERVES: 1 to 2
TIME: 5 minutes

1 packet frozen unsweetened acai puree (about 3½ ounces)
¾ cup frozen pineapple
1 cup spinach (fresh or frozen)
¾ cup unsweetened almond milk
2 tablespoons chia seeds
1 tablespoon almond butter
2 tablespoons collagen peptides (omit if vegan)

TOPPINGS (OPTIONAL)
Blueberries
Sliced almonds
Shredded unsweetened coconut
Cacao nibs

Add the acai, pineapple, spinach, and almond milk to a high-speed blender. Blend until well combined, then add the chia seeds, almond butter, and collagen peptides. Continue blending until very smooth.

Top, if desired, with blueberries, sliced almonds, shredded coconut, or cacao nibs for extra crunch and flavor. Serve immediately.

POWER PLATE LUNCH RECIPES

Spicy Lentil and Sweet Potato Salad with Vinaigrette

VF

SERVES: 1

TIME: 10 minutes

SALAD

2 cups fresh spinach

⅓ cup cubed roasted sweet potatoes

⅓ cup blueberries

¼ cup cooked lentils

1 tablespoon roasted pepitas

VINAIGRETTE

½ cup red wine vinegar

⅓ cup honey (or maple syrup or coconut nectar if vegan)

1 tablespoon adobo sauce

1 tablespoon fresh oregano

1 teaspoon cumin

1 teaspoon garlic powder

⅛ teaspoon black pepper, or to taste

1 cup extra-virgin olive oil

To make the salad, in a large bowl, combine the spinach, roasted sweet potato, blueberries, lentils, and pepitas.

To make the vinaigrette, in a high-speed blender or food processor, combine the vinegar, honey, 1 tablespoon of water, the adobo sauce, oregano, cumin, garlic powder, and pepper. Pulse until combined, then drizzle in the olive oil and blend until well emulsified. You'll end up with 2 cups of dressing, so save the extra for other salads or recipes.

Drizzle 1 to 2 tablespoons of the dressing over the salad before serving.

> TIP: Roast the sweet potatoes and cook the lentils ahead of time so the salad comes together quickly for a healthy lunch.

Quinoa Pasta with Pan-Seared Chicken and Creamy Avocado Spinach Sauce

SERVES: 2

TIME: 15 minutes

1 cup quinoa pasta

1 avocado, peeled and pitted

¼ cup + 1 teaspoon extra-virgin olive oil

2 tablespoons fresh lime juice

1 tablespoon fresh cilantro

½ cup fresh spinach

¼ teaspoon black pepper

2 chicken breasts

Cook the quinoa pasta according to the package directions; be careful not to overcook.

While the pasta is cooking, add the avocado, ¼ cup of the olive oil, the lime juice, cilantro, spinach, and black pepper to a high-speed blender. Blend on high until well combined. Set aside.

If the chicken breasts are extra thick, slice them into thinner cuts. In a medium pan, heat the remaining teaspoon of olive oil over medium-high heat until hot. Add the chicken to the pan and let cook for 5 minutes, then flip once and continue cooking for another 5 to 7 minutes, or until cooked all the way through (the internal temperature of the chicken should be 165ºF). Divide the quinoa pasta into two serving bowls, then top with the chicken and the avocado sauce to serve.

Savory Steel-Cut Oats with Fried Egg

SERVES: 4
TIME: 10 minutes, plus overnight in the slow cooker

- 2 cups steel-cut oats
- 4 eggs
- 2 tablespoons olive oil, divided
- 1 cup shredded Brussels sprouts
- 1 avocado, sliced
- ¼ teaspoon black pepper

Prepare the steel-cut oats the night before by adding the oats and 8 cups of water to a slow cooker and cooking on low for 8 hours. In the morning, fry the eggs in 1 tablespoon of olive oil, then sauté the Brussels sprouts in the remaining tablespoon of olive oil. Divide the oatmeal into four serving dishes and top each with a fried egg, Brussels sprouts, sliced avocado, and pepper to serve.

TIP: To save time, buy pre-shredded Brussels sprouts at the grocery store.

Roasted Butternut Squash Pecan Quinoa Salad

VF

SERVES: 4

TIME: 25 minutes

1 medium butternut squash, peeled and cubed

Extra-virgin olive oil

Salt and black pepper

1 cup pecan halves

½ cup coarsely chopped walnuts

2 tablespoons honey (or maple syrup or coconut nectar if vegan)

1 cup quinoa, rinsed and strained

¼ cup apple cider vinegar

⅛ teaspoon ground cinnamon

⅛ teaspoon ground ginger

1 cup sliced scallions

2 green apples, peeled and diced

Preheat the oven to 400ºF. Line two baking sheets with parchment paper.

Place the butternut squash cubes in a medium bowl, and toss with 1 tablespoon of olive oil. Arrange the squash on one of the prepared baking sheets in a single layer. Bake for 20 minutes, stirring occasionally.

In a small bowl, toss the pecans and walnuts with 1 teaspoon of olive oil and 1 tablespoon of the honey. Arrange the nut mixture on the other prepared baking sheet. Bake in the oven on a separate rack during the last 5 to 10 minutes, or until toasted, while the butternut squash is roasting.

Meanwhile, cook the quinoa according to the package directions. Set aside.

To make the dressing, in a small bowl, whisk together the vinegar, ¼ cup of olive oil, the remaining tablespoon of honey, the cinnamon, and the ground ginger. (Alternatively, put them in a jar with a lid and shake vigorously.)

In a large mixing bowl, place the roasted butternut squash, nuts, quinoa, scallions, and apples. Pour in the dressing and toss gently until combined. Season with salt and pepper to taste. Serve immediately.

Lentil Pasta with Butternut Squash "Cheesy" Sauce

VF

SERVES: 2

TIME: 30 minutes

1 cup lentil pasta

2 cups peeled and diced butternut squash

¼ cup unsweetened almond milk

2 tablespoons extra-virgin olive oil

1 teaspoon onion powder

½ teaspoon garlic powder

¼ cup nutritional yeast

1 tablespoon fresh lemon juice

Cook the lentil pasta according to the package directions; be careful not to overcook.

Boil or roast the butternut squash at 400°F for 10 to 20 minutes, until soft. Add the cooked butternut squash to a high-speed blender or food processor, along with the almond milk, olive oil, onion powder, garlic powder, nutritional yeast, and lemon juice, and blend on high until well combined.

Top the lentil pasta with the butternut squash sauce and serve immediately.

Barley Salad with Lemony Kale Pesto

VF

SERVES: 4

TIME: 35 minutes

1 cup pearled barley
½ cup extra-virgin olive oil
½ cup currants
⅛ teaspoon salt
1 tablespoon minced shallot
2 tablespoons coarsely chopped walnuts
3 to 4 handfuls kale, stems removed and leaves chopped
1 tablespoon fresh lemon juice

In a medium saucepan, cook the barley in boiling water until al dente, about 30 minutes. Drain thoroughly and let cool.

In a small skillet, heat 1 teaspoon of the olive oil. Cook the currants, salt, and shallot over medium heat until the shallot is golden, about 3 minutes. Add to the barley along with the walnuts.

In a food processor, add two-thirds of the kale leaves and the lemon juice. Process until the kale is thoroughly chopped.

With the machine on, slowly drizzle in the remaining olive oil until smooth. Add the kale pesto to the barley mixture along with the remaining kale leaves and toss to combine. Serve immediately.

Quinoa, Tempeh, and Roasted Veggie Salad with Walnut Dressing

VF

SERVES: 4

TIME: 40 minutes

1 cup quinoa, roasted and strained
Extra-virgin olive oil
16 ounces tempeh, thinly sliced into strips
2 zucchini, sliced into rounds
½ pound shiitake mushrooms, stemmed
½ pound asparagus, ends removed
1 red onion, sliced

DRESSING
1 cup walnuts
1 shallot, finely chopped
1 teaspoon fresh thyme leaves
½ teaspoon lemon zest
2 tablespoons fresh lemon juice
¼ teaspoon black pepper
¼ cup chopped fresh chives

Preheat the oven to 400ºF. Line a baking sheet with parchment paper or foil.

Cook the quinoa according to the package directions. Transfer the cooked quinoa to a large bowl.

Heat 1 tablespoon olive oil in a large skillet over medium-high heat. Add the tempeh slices and cook for 2 to 3 minutes, then flip and cook for another 2 minutes.

Spread the zucchini, mushrooms, asparagus, and onion onto the prepared baking sheet and lightly brush with olive oil. Roast for 20 minutes until nice and browned. Remove the vegetables from the oven and lower the heat to 350ºF.

To make the dressing, place the walnuts onto a baking sheet and toast until fragrant, about 10 minutes. Let the walnuts cool completely. Transfer them to a food processor. Add the shallot, thyme, lemon zest, 1 tablespoon of the lemon juice, ½ cup olive oil, and the pepper. Pulse until the nuts are coarsely chopped.

Cut the roasted vegetables into bite-size pieces and add to the quinoa, along with the walnut dressing, chives, and the remaining 1 tablespoon lemon juice, and stir until incorporated. Top with the tempeh and toss again to coat. Serve warm.

Strawberry Spinach Salad with Tofu and Simple Dressing

VF

SERVES: 4

TIME: 15 minutes

10 ounces baby spinach

¼ red onion, sliced

2 cups strawberries, hulled and quartered

½ cup blueberries

½ avocado, thinly sliced

½ cup pecan halves

16 ounces tofu, crumbled

SIMPLE DRESSING

¼ cup extra-virgin olive oil

¼ cup white wine vinegar

1 tablespoon Dijon mustard

2 garlic cloves, minced

⅛ teaspoon salt

¼ teaspoon black pepper

In a large bowl, add the spinach, red onion, strawberries, blueberries, avocado, pecan halves, and crumbled tofu.

To make the dressing, in a mason jar, combine the olive oil, vinegar, mustard, garlic, salt, and pepper. Shake thoroughly. (Or add to a high-speed blender or food processor and blend until well combined.)

Pour the dressing over the salad and divide into four servings. Keep the dressing and salad separate if not serving immediately and store in the refrigerator.

TIP: Opt for unseasoned tofu and make it slightly crispy by searing it in a skillet.

Creamy Avocado Chicken Salad Wraps

SERVES: 4

TIME: 10 minutes

2 avocados, peeled and pitted

2 tablespoons fresh lime juice

Salt

2 cups cooked shredded chicken

⅓ cup diced red onion

¼ cup chopped fresh cilantro

1 tablespoon minced jalapeño, seeds removed

4 whole-wheat or brown rice wraps

In a large bowl, mash together the avocado, lime juice, and salt to taste. Add the shredded chicken, onion, cilantro, and jalapeño until well incorporated. Divide into four servings, then spread the chicken salad onto a wrap and fold up. Repeat for the remaining wraps.

Serve immediately or store in the refrigerator.

> TIP: To save time, buy a rotisserie chicken from your local grocery store. Discard the skin, then remove the chicken breast from the top and shred it into small pieces. You can save the dark meat for another meal and use the carcass to make homemade chicken bone broth, if desired.

Broiled Orange Teriyaki Salmon with Edamame and Quinoa

SERVES: 4

TIME: 1 hour 25 minutes

4 (6-ounce) wild-caught salmon fillets

¼ cup extra-virgin olive oil

1 tablespoon orange zest

Juice of 1 orange

¼ cup coconut aminos

1 tablespoon maple syrup

1 teaspoon garlic powder

1 teaspoon spicy mustard

2 cups edamame

1 cup quinoa, rinsed and strained

¼ cup fresh chopped cilantro

Place the salmon in a zip-top bag and add the olive oil, orange zest, orange juice, coconut aminos, maple syrup, garlic powder, and spicy mustard. Marinate for at least 1 hour in the refrigerator before broiling.

Steam the edamame according to the package instructions.

Cook the quinoa according to the package directions. Set aside.

When the salmon has finished marinating, turn the broiler on high. Place the salmon on a baking sheet and broil for 5 minutes, then flip and cook for another 5 minutes until it is cooked through.

Serve the salmon on top of the cooked edamame and quinoa and top with chopped cilantro. Serve immediately.

TIP: For fuller flavor, allow the salmon to marinate overnight and prepare the next day.

Shredded Brussels Sprouts and Kale Salad with Roasted Sweet Potatoes and Almond Butter Dressing

VF

SERVES: 4

TIME: 30 minutes

SALAD

⅓ cup pecan halves

2 medium-size sweet potatoes, peeled

Vegetable oil cooking spray

1 pound Brussels sprouts, shredded

1 bunch kale, stems removed, shredded

2 medium apples, chopped

ALMOND BUTTER DRESSING

3 tablespoons balsamic vinegar

1 tablespoon extra-virgin olive oil

2 tablespoons maple syrup

¼ cup almond butter

1½ tablespoons mustard

⅛ teaspoon salt

Preheat the oven to 300°F.

To make the salad, place the pecans on a baking sheet in a single layer. Roast for 10 to 15 minutes, until fragrant, then remove from the oven and let cool for a few minutes. Turn the oven up to 400°F.

Dice the sweet potatoes and spread on a baking sheet in a single layer. Lightly spray with vegetable oil cooking spray. Roast for about 20 minutes, remove from the oven, and let cool slightly.

In a large mixing bowl, combine the shredded Brussels sprouts, kale, apples, roasted pecans, and roasted sweet potatoes. Toss together.

To make the dressing, in a bowl, combine the vinegar, olive oil, maple syrup, almond butter, mustard, and salt and whisk together. (Or shake in a jar with a lid on.) Add 2 to 4 tablespoons of water as needed to thin it out. Toss the salad with the dressing and serve immediately.

> TIP: If you're meal prepping, roast the pecans and sweet potatoes ahead of time and keep the dressing and salad separate until ready to serve.

Quinoa-Stuffed Acorn Squash

VF

SERVES: 4

TIME: 35 minutes

2 acorn squashes

Extra-virgin olive oil

1 cup quinoa, rinsed and strained

1 onion, diced

1 garlic clove, minced

1 pound mushrooms, chopped (shiitake or button)

6 celery stalks, diced

2 teaspoons chopped fresh rosemary

⅛ teaspoon salt

½ teaspoon black pepper

1 tablespoon chopped fresh parsley

2 teaspoons freshly grated lemon zest

Preheat the oven to 375°F. Line a baking sheet with parchment paper or foil.

Cut each squash in half and scoop out the seeds. Rub a little olive oil on the inside of each squash and place face-down on the prepared baking sheet. Bake 30 minutes, until fork tender.

Meanwhile, cook the quinoa according to the package directions. Set aside.

Heat 1 tablespoon of olive oil in a skillet over medium-high heat. Add the onion and garlic and cook for 2 minutes, stirring occasionally. Add the mushrooms, celery, rosemary, salt, and pepper. Cook, stirring occasionally, for 5 minutes.

Transfer the vegetables to a large mixing bowl and add the quinoa. Stir to combine. Add the parsley and lemon zest and stir to combine. Spoon the quinoa filling into each half of the roasted acorn squash and serve immediately.

Tuna Salad Sandwich

SERVES: 4

TIME: 5 minutes

¼ cup plain Greek yogurt

1 teaspoon Dijon mustard

Juice of ½ lemon

⅛ teaspoon salt

⅛ teaspoon black pepper

1 (3-ounce) can wild-caught tuna, drained

1 celery stalk, diced

1 tablespoon chopped chives (optional)

1 cup baby spinach

8 slices Ezekiel bread (toasted, optional)

In a small bowl, combine the Greek yogurt, mustard, lemon juice, salt, and pepper. Set aside. In a separate bowl, combine the tuna, diced celery, and chives (if using). Add the Greek yogurt mixture and stir until well combined.

Layer spinach on 4 slices of the bread, then top with the tuna salad. Top with the remaining 4 slices of bread and serve.

Healthy Egg Salad Wrap

SERVES: 4

TIME: 35 minutes

8 eggs

4 cups ice cubes

½ cup Vegenaise or plain Greek yogurt

1 tablespoon Dijon mustard

2 teaspoons fresh lemon juice

1 teaspoon chopped fresh chives

1 tablespoon chopped scallion

1 teaspoon chopped fresh dill

⅛ teaspoon salt

¼ teaspoon black pepper

4 whole-wheat or brown rice wraps

Start by hard-boiling the eggs: Place the eggs in a large pot with enough water to cover them. Cover with a lid and bring the water to a boil over high heat. Once the water is boiling, shut off the heat and leave the eggs in the pot with the lid on for 10 minutes. Remove the eggs and place in a bowl with 4 cups of water and the ice. Let the eggs cool for 15 minutes and then remove the shells.

Roughly chop the hard-boiled eggs. In a mixing bowl, add the chopped eggs, Vegenaise (or Greek yogurt), Dijon mustard, lemon juice, chives, scallion, dill, salt, and black pepper. Mix together, tasting occasionally to adjust the seasonings as needed.

Use roughly ½ cup of the egg salad in each wrap and serve immediately. Store unused portions in the refrigerator.

> TIP: To save time, boil the eggs ahead of time—and do it in big batches!

Beet and Bean Burger

VF

SERVES: 6

TIME: 1 hour 15 minutes, plus at least 2 hours in the refrigerator

1 pound beets
½ cup brown rice
1 onion, diced
Extra-virgin olive oil
3 garlic cloves, minced
2 tablespoons apple cider vinegar
¼ cup old-fashioned oats
2 (15-ounce) cans black beans, drained and rinsed

2 teaspoons smoked paprika

2 teaspoons brown mustard

1 teaspoon ground cumin

½ teaspoon ground coriander

½ teaspoon dried thyme

⅛ teaspoon salt

Black pepper

1 egg (optional; omit if vegan)

6 whole-wheat hamburger buns or lettuce leaves

Preheat the oven to 400°F.

Wrap the beets loosely in aluminum foil and roast for 50 to 60 minutes, or until tender. Set aside to cool.

Meanwhile, add 1¼ cups of water to a pot and bring to a boil over high heat. Add the rice and simmer over medium heat for 35 to 40 minutes, until cooked through. Set aside to cool.

In the meantime, sauté the onion in a skillet over medium-high heat with 1 teaspoon of olive oil. Stir occasionally until golden brown, 10 to 12 minutes. Add the garlic at the end and cook until fragrant, about 30 seconds. Pour in the vinegar and scrape any crust left from the onions on the bottom of the pan. Simmer until the vinegar has mostly evaporated and the pan is dry. Set aside from the heat to let cool.

Pulverize the oats in a food processor until they are reduced to a flour. Transfer to a small bowl. Add the black beans to the food processor and pulse until the beans are roughly chopped. Transfer the chopped beans to a large mixing bowl.

Remove the skin from the roasted beets. Grate the beets using a large cheese grater, or roughly chop them into small chunks. Place the beets in a mesh strainer set over the sink or a bowl, and squeeze as much liquid out as possible.

Transfer the beets, cooked rice, and onions to the mixing bowl with the beans. Add 1 tablespoon of olive oil, the smoked paprika, brown mustard, cumin, coriander, thyme, salt, and pepper to taste. Whisk the egg, if using, and add it along with the ground oats. Continue mixing until well incorporated. Cover the mixture and place in the refrigerator for at least 2 hours or overnight.

When ready to cook, remove the mixture from the refrigerator. Form 6 patties using your hands. Heat a large skillet over medium-high heat and add enough olive oil to lightly cover the bottom. Cook each patty for 2 minutes on one side, then flip and cook another 2 minutes.

Cover the skillet with a lid and reduce the heat to medium-low and continue cooking for another 4 minutes, until the burgers are heated through. Serve them on whole-wheat hamburger buns or lettuce leaves.

TIP: Whip up this dish in a flash by cooking the beets ahead of time and using a steamable bag of brown rice—these tricks will cut your prep time by an hour!

Honey Sesame Seared Salmon with Spicy Cabbage Slaw

SERVES: 4
TIME: 1 hour 15 minutes

SALMON

¼ cup coconut aminos

¼ cup sesame oil

Juice of 1 lemon

2 tablespoons honey

1 teaspoon ground ginger

4 (8-ounce) wild-caught salmon fillets

1 tablespoon coconut oil

1 tablespoon sesame seeds

1 scallion, sliced

SPICY CABBAGE SLAW

½ head cabbage, thinly sliced

¼ cup thinly sliced red onion

1 cup shredded carrots

2 garlic cloves, minced

2 tablespoons chopped fresh cilantro (optional)

2 tablespoons chopped fresh parsley

¼ cup apple cider vinegar

¼ cup extra-virgin olive oil

Juice of ½ lemon

⅛ teaspoon salt

¼ teaspoon garlic powder

⅛ teaspoon onion powder

¼ teaspoon red pepper flakes

To make the salmon, in a bowl, combine the coconut aminos, sesame oil, lemon juice, honey, and ground ginger and whisk until smooth. Place the salmon in a zip-top storage bag or glass dish and cover in the marinade. Let marinate for at least 1 hour, or overnight if possible.

In a large skillet, heat the coconut oil over medium-high heat. Place the salmon in the skillet skin side down. Cook for 2 to 3 minutes, then turn the salmon fillets over. Pour the remaining marinade in the skillet. Cook on the second side for 3 to 5 minutes, until the salmon easily flakes with a fork. Transfer the salmon to plates and sprinkle the fillets with the sesame seeds and scallion.

Prepare the cabbage slaw: In a large mixing bowl, combine the cabbage, red onion, carrots, garlic, cilantro (if using), and parsley. In a small bowl, whisk together the vinegar, olive oil, lemon juice, salt, garlic powder, onion powder, and red pepper flakes. Add the dressing to the slaw vegetables and stir together until well combined. Serve the slaw alongside the salmon.

Curry Chicken Lettuce Wraps

SERVES: 2

TIME: 15 minutes

CURRY CHICKEN
1 tablespoon extra-virgin olive oil
1 garlic clove, minced
1 scallion, chopped
1 teaspoon ground turmeric
6 fresh mint leaves, chopped
1 teaspoon ground cumin
1 tablespoon sesame seeds
1 tablespoon flaxseeds
1 teaspoon red pepper flakes
2 chicken breasts, cooked and shredded

AVOCADO SALAD
1 avocado, peeled, pitted, and sliced
1 teaspoon fresh lime juice
1 garlic clove, minced
1 scallion, chopped
12 fresh basil leaves, chiffonade (cut into long, thin strips)

4 to 8 large lettuce leaves

To make the curry chicken, in a large skillet, heat the olive oil over medium heat. Sauté the garlic and scallion for 1 to 3 minutes, or under tender, then add the turmeric, mint leaves, cumin, sesame seeds, flaxseeds, and red pepper flakes and stir until a thick paste is formed. Add the shredded chicken and stir until the chicken is well coated. Remove from the heat and set aside.

To make the avocado salad, mix together the avocado, lime juice, garlic, scallion, and basil.

Fill the lettuce leaves with the chicken curry mixture, then top with avocado salad. Serve immediately.

Chicken Enchilada Cauliflower Rice Bowl

SERVES: 4
TIME: 30 minutes

ENCHILADA CHICKEN
2 teaspoons chili powder
1 cup low-sodium red enchilada sauce
4 chicken breasts

CAULIFLOWER RICE
1 head cauliflower, chopped into florets
⅛ teaspoon salt
1 teaspoon chili powder
¼ teaspoon garlic powder
Juice of 1 lime
2 tablespoons chopped fresh cilantro

TOPPINGS
Black olives, sliced
Diced avocado
Chopped fresh cilantro
Diced tomato

To make the enchilada chicken, in a deep pot, combine the chili powder and red enchilada sauce and bring to a boil over medium-high heat. Lower the heat to medium-low and place the chicken breasts in the sauce, making sure they are mostly covered by the sauce. Place a lid over the pot and cook for 15 to 20 minutes, until the chicken is cooked through.

Once the chicken is done, shred it with two forks and stir it back into the sauce.

To make the cauliflower rice, pulse the cauliflower florets in a food processor until it is the size of rice. Heat a skillet over medium-high heat and add the cauliflower rice, salt, chili powder, and garlic powder. Sauté for a few minutes, stirring occasionally. Stir in the lime juice and cilantro, cooking for 1 more minute.

To serve, divide the cauliflower rice into four serving bowls, then add the enchilada chicken and sauce. Top with olives, avocado, cilantro, and tomatoes.

Turkey Meatballs with Zucchini Noodles and Avocado Sauce

SERVES: 4 (12 to 15 meatballs)
TIME: 40 minutes

1 pound lean ground turkey
⅛ teaspoon salt
½ teaspoon black pepper
1 teaspoon garlic powder
1 teaspoon onion powder
¼ cup coconut flour
½ red onion, minced
2 to 3 sprigs fresh parsley, minced
2 eggs
2 large zucchini

AVOCADO SAUCE

2 avocados, peeled and pitted

½ onion, roughly chopped

2 garlic cloves

Juice of ½ lime

¼ cup chopped fresh parsley or cilantro

¼ to ½ cup water

⅛ teaspoon salt

½ teaspoon black pepper

Preheat the oven to 375°F. Line a baking sheet with parchment paper and set aside.

Place the ground turkey in a large bowl.

In a separate bowl, mix together the salt, black pepper, garlic powder, onion powder, coconut flour, minced onion, and minced parsley. Add the spice mixture to the ground turkey and work with your hands to combine it all.

Whisk the eggs together. Top the turkey mixture with the eggs and continue mixing with your hands until well combined. Form into 12 to 15 meatballs, space them out evenly on the prepared baking sheet, and bake for 30 to 35 minutes, until golden brown on the outside.

Meanwhile, cut the zucchini into noodles using a spiralizer or a vegetable peeler.

To make the avocado sauce, combine the avocados, onion, garlic, lime juice, parsley, and water in a high-speed blender until smooth and creamy. Add the salt and pepper and blend again.

Divide the zucchini noodles into four serving bowls and top with the meatballs and avocado sauce. Serve immediately.

Slow-Cooker Beef with Broccoli

SERVES: 4

TIME: 10 minutes, plus up to 6 hours in the slow cooker

1¼ pounds beef sirloin or other lean cut of steak

1 onion, diced

2 tablespoons minced fresh ginger

2 garlic cloves, minced

6 tablespoons coconut aminos

2 teaspoons tapioca or arrowroot starch

2 tablespoons sesame oil

½ tablespoon fish sauce (optional)

4 cups chopped broccoli

4 cups cauliflower rice

2 scallions, chopped

Sesame seeds

Slice the beef into very thin slices, about ¼-inch strips. Add the sliced beef into a slow cooker, along with the onion, ginger, and garlic.

In a small bowl, whisk together the coconut aminos, 2 tablespoons water, and tapioca or arrowroot starch. Once combined, whisk in the sesame oil and fish sauce (if using). Pour the sauce in the slow cooker and stir until the beef and vegetables are coated. Cook in the slow cooker on low for 4 to 6 hours or on high for 2 to 3 hours.

Add the broccoli to the slow cooker and stir until coated. Continue cooking for another 30 minutes on high. If desired, add the cauliflower rice to the mixture as well and let cook with the beef and broccoli. Alternatively, in a skillet, combine ¼ cup of water with the cauliflower rice and cover and steam for 7 to 10 minutes, stirring occasionally.

If you've steamed the cauliflower rice separately, divide it into four serving bowls and top with the beef and broccoli. Sprinkle with the scallions and sesame seeds to serve.

Pesto Whitefish Packets with Veggies

SERVES: 2

TIME: 45 minutes

2 bell peppers, cored, seeded, and thinly sliced

2 zucchini, thinly sliced

2 (6-ounce) whitefish fillets, such as cod, tilapia, flounder, halibut, or mahimahi

HOMEMADE PESTO

1 cup packed fresh basil

¼ cup chopped fresh parsley

1 tablespoon walnuts

1 garlic clove

1 tablespoon fresh lemon juice

¼ cup extra-virgin olive oil, plus more as needed

⅛ teaspoon salt

¼ teaspoon black pepper

Preheat the oven to 400°F.

Place two large squares of foil on top of a baking sheet. Create a bed of bell pepper and zucchini slices in each square. Place one fillet on top of each bed of vegetables.

To make the pesto, in a food processor, add the basil, parsley, walnuts, garlic, and lemon juice. Pulse a few times, then slowly drizzle in the olive oil to create pesto. Add more oil if the pesto is too thick. Add the salt and pepper, and pulse a few more times.

Divide the pesto mixture between the two foil packs and place it on top of the fish fillets and vegetables. Fold the foil around the fish and vegetables until closed, leaving a small opening for steam to escape. Bake for 12 to 15 minutes, until the fish is opaque and is easily flaked with a fork. Be careful of steam when opening the foil packets.

Serve immediately.

> TIP: Experiment with different varieties of whitefish and see which ones your taste buds prefer. While they won't differ drastically in taste or texture, there are slight nuances among each kind.

Low-Carb Chicken Pad Thai with Vegetable Noodles

SERVES: 4
TIME: 20 minutes

2 zucchini

1 tablespoon extra-virgin olive oil

1 pound chicken breasts, cut into 1-inch chunks

⅛ teaspoon salt

Black pepper

1 cup shredded carrots

½ red onion, diced

3 bell peppers (orange, red, and yellow), diced

3 scallions, thinly sliced

PAD THAI SAUCE

½ cup almond butter or natural peanut butter

2 tablespoons honey

1 tablespoon sesame oil

2 tablespoons coconut aminos

2 garlic cloves, minced

1 teaspoon ground ginger

1 tablespoon rice wine vinegar

2 tablespoons fresh lime juice

TOPPINGS

Crushed peanuts

Fresh basil

Lime wedges

Peel or spiralize the zucchini into noodles and set aside.

Heat the olive oil in a large skillet over medium-high heat. Add the chicken breast chunks and sauté for 3 to 4 minutes on each side until browned and cooked through. Season with the salt and black pepper to taste. Remove the cooked chicken from the pan and set aside.

Spray the same pan with vegetable oil cooking spray and add the carrots, red onion, bell peppers, and scallions. Sauté over medium-high heat. Stir frequently, until the onions are translucent and the vegetables begin to soften.

To make the sauce, in a medium bowl, combine the nut butter, honey, sesame oil, coconut aminos, garlic, ginger, rice wine vinegar, and lime juice. Add water a tablespoon at a time if needed to thin the sauce out.

Add the cooked chicken and zucchini noodles to the skillet with the cooked vegetables and toss together. Cook on low until everything is heated.

Serve and garnish with peanuts, basil, and lime wedges.

Chicken Alfredo Spaghetti Squash

SERVES: 4

TIME: 2 hours

1 pound chicken breasts, sliced
Juice of ½ lemon
2 teaspoons garlic powder
¼ teaspoon salt
1 spaghetti squash
2 tablespoons coconut oil
1 medium head cauliflower, chopped
¼ cup canned coconut milk
¼ cup low-sodium chicken broth
1 tablespoon extra-virgin olive oil
Fresh basil, chopped

Season the chicken breast slices with lemon juice, 1 teaspoon of the garlic powder, and ⅛ teaspoon of the salt, and allow to marinate in the refrigerator for an hour. Preheat the oven to 400°F.

Slice the squash in half lengthwise and scoop out the seeds. Place the squash cut-side down in a roasting pan or 9 × 13-inch baking dish. Bake for 30 to 40 minutes, until easily pierced with a fork and strands come out easily.

Heat the coconut oil in a skillet over medium-high heat. Add the chicken and let cook for 5 to 7 minutes, before flipping over once and cooking for another 5 minutes, or until cooked through. Chicken should be at least 165°F internally when done. Set the chicken aside.

To make the Alfredo sauce, add the cauliflower to a medium pot and fill the pot about two-thirds with water. Bring to a simmer over medium heat and cook for 8 to 10 minutes, until the cauliflower is soft. Strain the cauliflower and let it cool.

In a high-speed blender or food processor, blend the cauliflower with the coconut milk, chicken broth, olive oil, the remaining teaspoon of garlic powder, and the remaining ⅛ teaspoon of salt until smooth.

Scoop the spaghetti squash strands out into a large dish. Top with the sauce, reserving some for topping at the end. Add the sliced chicken, fresh basil, and remaining sauce. Serve immediately.

> TIP: This dish is easy to make vegetarian—just omit the chicken and use vegetable broth.

Crunchy Coconut and Kale Salmon

SERVES: 2

TIME: 20 minutes

SWEET AND SPICY SAUCE

2 tablespoons coconut aminos

1½ tablespoons rice wine vinegar

1 tablespoon almond butter

1 tablespoon maple syrup (optional)

1 tablespoon sesame oil

1 teaspoon hot sauce

1 teaspoon minced fresh ginger or ¼ teaspoon ground ginger

1 teaspoon garlic powder

SALMON

2 tablespoons coconut oil (solid)

2 (6-ounce) wild-caught salmon fillets

½ cup unsweetened coconut flakes

7 to 8 lacinato kale leaves, stalks removed, thinly sliced

To make the sweet and spicy sauce, in a glass jar with a lid, combine the coconut aminos, rice wine vinegar, almond butter, maple syrup (if using), sesame oil, hot sauce, ginger, and garlic powder. Shake vigorously until well mixed.

To make the salmon, in a large saucepan, melt the coconut oil over medium heat. Place the salmon (skin side up if it is still on) into the pan. Cook the salmon for 5 minutes. Turn it over and cook for 30 seconds on the other side. Pour a few tablespoons of the sauce over the salmon and continue cooking. Stir in the shredded coconut and stir occasionally.

Add the kale, along with a few more tablespoons of the sauce, and cook until the leaves are wilted and have absorbed much of the sauce. Once the salmon flakes easily with a fork, it is ready to serve—2 to 3 more minutes.

To serve, divide among two serving plates and drizzle any remaining sauce on top of each dish.

> TIP: Lacinato kale is sturdier and has a lighter flavor than green kale. It has a nice crunchy texture when sautéed or roasted as well!

Chicken Zoodle Soup

SERVES: 6

TIME: 30 minutes

2 tablespoons extra-virgin olive oil

1 pound chicken breasts, cut into 1-inch pieces

⅛ teaspoon salt

¼ teaspoon black pepper

3 garlic cloves, minced

1 onion, diced

3 carrots, sliced

2 celery stalks, diced

½ teaspoon dried thyme

¼ teaspoon dried rosemary

4 cups low-sodium chicken broth

3 to 5 zucchini (about 1 pound), spiralized

2 tablespoons fresh lemon juice

1 sprig fresh rosemary, chopped (optional)

2 tablespoons chopped fresh parsley (optional)

In a large stockpot, heat 1 tablespoon of the olive oil over medium heat. Season the chicken with the salt and pepper. Add the chicken to the stockpot and cook, stirring occasionally, until browned, 2 to 3 minutes. Remove the chicken and set aside.

Add the remaining tablespoon of olive oil, the garlic, onion, carrots, and celery to the stockpot. Cook, stirring occasionally, until tender, 3 to 4 minutes. Stir in the dried thyme and rosemary until fragrant, about 1 minute.

Add the chicken broth and 2 cups of water to the stockpot and bring to a boil over high heat. Stir in the zucchini noodles and chicken. Reduce the heat to medium and simmer until the zucchini is tender, 3 to 5 minutes. Stir in the lemon juice.

Serve immediately, garnishing with fresh rosemary and parsley, if desired.

Cauliflower Crust BBQ Pizza

SERVES: 2
TIME: 20 minutes

1 pre-made cauliflower pizza crust
¼ cup low-sugar barbecue sauce
1 cup cooked shredded chicken
¼ cup shredded mozzarella cheese
½ cup diced red onion
2 tablespoons sliced jalapeños
2 tablespoons chopped fresh cilantro (optional)
2 tablespoons crushed peanuts

Preheat the oven to 400°F.

Cook just the crust—no toppings—according to the package instructions, and flip halfway through, once it starts to brown on the bottom. Let cool.

Top the crust with barbecue sauce, chicken, mozzarella, red onion, and jalapeños. Place back in the oven and broil for 5 to 10 minutes, until the cheese is melted. Top with cilantro (if using) and crushed peanuts and serve immediately.

TIP: Be careful of the carbohydrate content when using a pre-made cauliflower crust. I use the Cali'flour brand's Cali'Lite collection specifically because it has only 6 grams of carbs in the whole crust.

Cauli-Fried Rice with Eggs and Veggies

SERVES: 4

TIME: 30 minutes

1 medium head cauliflower

3 eggs

Vegetable oil cooking spray

1 tablespoon sesame oil

¼ teaspoon salt

½ onion, diced

5 scallions, white and green parts sliced and separated

½ cup frozen peas

½ cup shredded carrots

2 garlic cloves, minced

3 tablespoons coconut aminos

1 to 2 teaspoons hot sauce (optional)

Remove the core and chop the cauliflower into florets. Place the florets into a food processor and pulse until it resembles rice.

In a small bowl, whisk the eggs together. Spray a large skillet with vegetable oil cooking spray and heat the skillet over medium-high heat. Add the eggs and cook until set, then set aside. Add the sesame oil to the skillet, then add the salt, onion, the white parts of the scallions, the peas, carrots, and garlic. Sauté for a few minutes, until softened.

Add the cauliflower rice and coconut aminos to the skillet. Cook for 5 to 6 minutes, stirring occasionally. The cauliflower should be crispy on the outside and tender on the inside. Remove from the heat and top with the cooked egg and the green parts of the scallions.

Top with the hot sauce, if desired, and serve immediately.

TIP: Buy frozen cauliflower rice and shredded carrots to shave minutes off preparing this recipe.

Steak Salad with Rosemary Olive Oil Dressing

SERVES: 4

TIME: 30 minutes, plus at least several hours to marinate

¼ cup balsamic vinegar

¼ cup extra-virgin olive oil

2 teaspoons fresh lemon juice

1 teaspoon chopped fresh rosemary

⅛ teaspoon salt

⅛ teaspoon black pepper

¾ pound lean steak such as top sirloin, sirloin tip, or filet

3 cups of arugula

½ cup sliced radishes or shredded carrots

1 zucchini, diced

1 avocado, diced

¼ red onion, thinly sliced

To make the dressing, in a medium bowl, whisk together the balsamic vinegar, olive oil, lemon juice, rosemary, salt, and pepper.

Place the steak in a shallow dish or zip-top bag. Pour ¼ cup of the dressing over the steak and let it marinate in the refrigerator for at least several hours, up to overnight.

Once it has marinated, drain the steak and discard the marinade. Sear the steak in a skillet on high heat or broil it in the oven on high for 6 to 8 minutes on each side. Let stand for 5 minutes before slicing.

In a large mixing bowl, combine the arugula, radishes, zucchini, avocado, and onion and toss together. To serve, divide the salad among four serving bowls and top with the steak and remaining dressing.

TIP: Just a general PSA that a "medium" steak should have an internal temperature of 160°F.

Lettuce Wrap Street Tacos

SERVES: 4
TIME: 15 minutes

1 pound lean steak such as sirloin, strip, or filet
Vegetable oil cooking spray
⅛ teaspoon salt
¼ teaspoon black pepper
1 head Bibb or butter lettuce, separated into leaves
½ onion, chopped
1 avocado, diced
¼ cup chopped fresh cilantro (optional)
1 lime, quartered

Cut the steak into bite-size pieces. Spray a skillet lightly with vegetable oil cooking spray and set over medium-high heat. Season the steak with the salt and pepper, then sear the steak on both sides according to the degree of doneness you desire.

Fill the lettuce leaves with the cooked steak. Top the tacos with the onion, avocado, and cilantro (if using), then squeeze lime juice over the top. Serve immediately.

Salmon and Scallops Salad

SERVES: 2

TIME: 10 minutes

Vegetable oil cooking spray

2 (6-ounce) wild-caught salmon fillets

4 to 6 large scallops, thawed from frozen or fresh

⅛ teaspoon salt

⅛ teaspoon cayenne pepper

⅛ teaspoon garlic powder

1 (16-ounce) package frozen stir-fry vegetables

2 cups sliced mushrooms (shiitake or button)

1 cup halved cherry tomatoes

4 handfuls mixed spring greens

2 tablespoons sugar-free Green Goddess dressing, such as Tessemae's

Spray a skillet with vegetable oil cooking spray and heat over high heat. Add the salmon fillets and scallops, then sprinkle with the salt, cayenne pepper, and garlic powder. Sear until the fillets and scallops are crispy on the outside, then flip and cook until crispy on the other side.

Meanwhile, steam the bag of stir-fry veggies in the microwave according to the package directions. In a small skillet, sauté the mushrooms and cherry tomatoes in a small amount of water over high heat until tender.

To serve, divide the mixed greens between two serving bowls and top with the salmon, scallops, and all of the veggies. Drizzle with the Green Goddess dressing.

> TIP: Anytime I make seafood or fish that can create a fishy smell in my house, I cook them outside on an electric skillet.

Szechuan Eggplant

VF

SERVES: 4 to 6

TIME: 30 minutes

1 tablespoon sesame oil

1 eggplant, peeled and cut into 1-inch cubes

1 onion, chopped

1 red bell pepper, seeded and chopped

¼ cup spicy Szechuan sauce

2 tablespoons coconut aminos

⅓ cup chopped raw cashews

2 (10-ounce) packages of riced cauliflower, microwaved from frozen

In a frying pan or wok, heat the sesame oil on medium heat. Add the eggplant, onion, and bell pepper. Sauté for 2 to 3 minutes, stirring frequently, or until the vegetables are soft.

Add the Szechuan sauce, coconut aminos, and cashews. Combine well until the vegetables are coated with sauce.

Serve over cauliflower rice.

Quick and Easy Black Bean Enchiladas

VF

SERVES: 4

TIME: 25 minutes

1 (15-ounce) can black beans, drained and rinsed
1 (4-ounce) can green chiles, drained
Vegetable oil cooking spray
8 cauliflower tortillas
1 (10-ounce) can low-sodium red enchilada sauce
3 scallions, chopped

Preheat the oven to 350ºF.

In a small microwavable dish, combine the beans and chiles. Microwave the mixture for 3 to 4 minutes or until heated through.

Spray a large glass baking dish with vegetable oil cooking spray. Arrange the tortillas in 1 layer in the prepared dish. Spoon the bean/chile mixture evenly in each tortilla, and roll the tortillas burrito-style. Pour enchilada sauce over the tortillas. Place in the oven and heat for 15 minutes.

Sprinkle the chopped scallions over the enchiladas prior to serving.

Stuffed Poblano Peppers

VF

SERVES: 4 to 6

TIME: 45 minutes

Vegetable oil cooking spray

6 large poblano peppers

2½ tablespoons extra-virgin olive oil

1 medium onion, chopped

1 cup chopped mushrooms (shiitake or button)

1 small zucchini, cubed

1 cup cauliflower rice, microwaved from frozen

¾ cup tomato puree

Salt and black pepper

¼ teaspoon cayenne pepper

Vegan cheese, shredded

Preheat the oven to 400°F. Spray a 9 × 13-inch baking dish with vegetable oil cooking spray and set aside.

Cut off the tops of the peppers and scoop out the seeds. Set aside.

In a large saucepan, heat the olive oil. Add the onion and sauté until soft, 2 to 3 minutes. Add the mushrooms and cook for an additional 5 to 6 minutes. Add the zucchini and cook for 5 minutes.

Remove from the heat. Stir in the cauliflower rice, tomato puree, salt and pepper to taste, and the cayenne.

Divide the mixture among the peppers. Place the stuffed peppers in the prepared baking dish. Bake for 20 minutes or until the peppers are soft.

Sprinkle generously with vegan cheese and serve.

POWER SNACKS, TREATS, AND SMOOTHIES

Note: Most of these recipes should be eaten prior to 4 p.m. because of their starchy carb content.

Peanut Butter Energy Balls

VF

SERVES: 18 balls or 3 balls per serving

TIME: 30 minutes

1¼ cups old-fashioned oats

1 tablespoon chia seeds

1 tablespoon flaxseeds

½ cup natural peanut butter (or other nut butter if you have a peanut allergy)

⅓ cup honey (or maple syrup or coconut nectar if vegan)

1 teaspoon vanilla extract

⅛ teaspoon salt (optional)

½ cup dark chocolate chips

In a large mixing bowl, add the oats, chia seeds, flaxseed, peanut butter, honey, vanilla extract, and salt (if using). Mix together until well incorporated. Fold in the chocolate chips.

Refrigerate the dough for 20 to 30 minutes. Remove from the refrigerator and scoop the dough into roughly 1-inch balls.

Store in the refrigerator or freezer. Thaw prior to serving.

Black Bean Brownies

SERVES: 12

TIME: 45 minutes

Vegetable oil cooking spray

1 (15-ounce) can black beans, drained and rinsed

3 eggs

⅓ cup coconut oil, melted

¼ cup unsweetened cocoa powder

2 teaspoons vanilla extract

¾ cup coconut sugar

½ cup dark chocolate chips

Preheat the oven to 350°F.

Spray an 8 × 8-inch or 9 × 9-inch baking dish with vegetable oil cooking spray and set aside.

In a high-speed blender or food processor, combine the black beans, eggs, melted coconut oil, cocoa powder, vanilla extract, and coconut sugar. Blend on high until the black beans are smooth. Pour into the prepared baking dish and top with the chocolate chips.

Bake for 40 minutes or until set and a toothpick inserted into the center comes out clean. Let cool before cutting into 12 bars. Store in the refrigerator.

Healthy Banana Nut Bread

SERVES: 10

TIME: 40 minutes

Vegetable oil cooking spray (optional)

1¾ cups mashed banana (about 3 ripe bananas)

½ cup chopped walnuts

2 cups old-fashioned oats

½ teaspoon ground cinnamon

¼ cup maple syrup

2 eggs

1 teaspoon baking powder

Preheat the oven to 350ºF. Line a standard loaf pan with parchment paper or spray with vegetable oil cooking spray.

In a large mixing bowl, mix the banana, walnuts, oats, cinnamon, maple syrup, eggs, and baking powder until well combined. Pour the batter into the prepared loaf pan.

Bake for 30 to 35 minutes until cooked through. Test for doneness by piercing the bread with a toothpick, and if it comes out clean, the bread is done. Let cool slightly before slicing and serving.

Banana Ice Cream

VF

SERVES: 4

TIME: 10 minutes

4 bananas, peeled, sliced, and frozen

¼ cup unsweetened almond milk

½ cup natural peanut butter (or other nut butter if you're allergic to peanuts)

In a high-speed blender or food processor, combine the frozen bananas, almond milk, and peanut butter. Process or blend until smooth and creamy, adding more liquid if needed to facilitate blending. Serve immediately.

Erin's Famous Beet Juice

VF

SERVES: 8 to 10

TIME: 10 minutes

2 bunches raw beets

3 lemons

1 inch of raw ginger

Without peeling any of the ingredients, throw them all into a juicer and turn it on high. Once all your ingredients have been juiced, divide and store in small, airtight containers like mini mason jars and store in the refrigerator. These shots are good for up to three days.

TIP: I recommend drinking 3 ounces of beet juice twice a day—once in the morning and once prior to working out. Read more about the power of beet juice, and why I drink it every day, on page 100.

Beets and Tart Cherry Smoothie

VF

SERVES: 1

TIME: 5 minutes

1 cup unsweetened almond milk

1 cooked beet, cut into quarters

½ cup frozen pitted cherries, unsweetened

½ frozen banana

1 tablespoon almond butter

In a high-speed blender, combine the almond milk, beet, cherries, banana, and almond butter. Blend until smooth and creamy. Serve immediately.

TIP: You can boil or roast your own beets or buy store-bought cooked ones. If you use store-bought beets, make sure they have no added salt or other ingredients.

Creamy Avocado and Mint Smoothie

VF

SERVES: 2

TIME: 5 minutes

1 frozen banana

½ frozen avocado

½ cup frozen spinach

2 tablespoons hemp or chia seeds

½ to 1 cup unsweetened almond milk

3 or 4 fresh mint leaves

In a high-speed blender, combine the banana, avocado, spinach, hemp seeds, almond milk, and mint leaves and blend until smooth. Serve.

> TIP: Using frozen ingredients creates a thick, creamy smoothie—add more liquid as necessary to facilitate blending.

Pumpkin Protein Smoothie

VF
SERVES: 2
TIME: 5 minutes

8 ice cubes

1 banana

½ cup pumpkin puree

3 tablespoons unsweetened almond milk

¾ cup plain Greek yogurt (or almond yogurt if vegan)

½ teaspoon pumpkin pie spice

2 tablespoons collagen peptides (omit if vegan)

In a high-speed blender, combine the ice cubes, banana, pumpkin puree, almond milk, yogurt, pumpkin pie spice, and collagen peptides. Blend until smooth. Serve immediately.

Protein Berry Muffins

SERVES: 12
TIME: 35 minutes

Vegetable oil cooking spray (optional)

2 eggs

½ cup unsweetened applesauce

1 cup unsweetened almond milk

1 teaspoon vanilla extract

2 tablespoons flaxseeds

¼ cup collagen peptides

3 cups old-fashioned oats

1 teaspoon ground cinnamon

⅛ teaspoon salt

1 cup blueberries (fresh or frozen)

Preheat the oven to 350°F. Line a muffin tin with paper liners or lightly grease with vegetable oil cooking spray.

In a mixing bowl, whisk together the eggs, applesauce, almond milk, and vanilla.

In a separate large bowl, mix together the flaxseeds, collagen peptides, oats, cinnamon, and salt. Add the dry mixture to the wet mixture and mix until well combined. Fold in the blueberries.

Transfer the batter to the prepared muffin tin and fill each cup about three-quarters of the way full. Bake for 20 minutes or until cooked through and golden brown on top. Let cool slightly before removing from the muffin tin to serve.

Healthy Freezer Fudge

VF

SERVES: 12

TIME: 5 minutes, plus 1 hour in the freezer

1 cup almond butter

⅓ cup coconut oil, slightly melted

¼ cup unsweetened cocoa powder

3 tablespoons honey (or maple syrup or coconut nectar if vegan)

⅛ teaspoon salt

1 teaspoon vanilla extract

Line a freezer-safe container with a lid with plastic wrap or parchment paper.

In a medium bowl, mix together the almond butter, coconut oil, cocoa powder, honey, salt, and vanilla until very smooth and creamy. Transfer the mixture to the prepared container.

Place the fudge in the freezer for at least 1 hour to set. Remove from the freezer to cut into 12 pieces and serve. Store in the freezer after slicing.

Banana Oatmeal Cookies

SERVES: 12

TIME: 20 minutes

- 2 eggs
- 3 mashed bananas
- 1 cup peanut butter (or other nut butter if you are allergic to peanuts)
- 1 tablespoon vanilla extract
- 3 cups old-fashioned oats
- 1 teaspoon ground cinnamon
- ½ cup dark chocolate chips

Preheat the oven to 350ºF. Line a baking sheet with parchment paper.

In a large mixing bowl, whisk together the eggs, mashed bananas, peanut butter, and vanilla extract. Add the oats and cinnamon and stir until well combined. Fold in the chocolate chips.

Scoop out 1-inch balls of dough onto the prepared baking sheet. Bake for 15 minutes. Let cool slightly before serving.

Dessert Pizza

SERVES: 10

TIME: 15 minutes

2 cups walnuts
1½ cups dates, pitted
2 cups plain Greek yogurt
3 tablespoons honey
1 teaspoon vanilla extract
1 cup blueberries
1 cup raspberries
1 cup strawberries, sliced

In a food processor, blend the walnuts and pitted dates until a sticky dough forms. Press this "crust" into a 9 × 13-inch baking dish or round pizza pan.

For the topping, mix together the Greek yogurt, honey, and vanilla extract. Spread the yogurt mixture on top of the walnut crust almost to the edge. Place the berries on top of the yogurt. Slice and serve immediately. Store leftovers in the refrigerator.

Pumpkin Bars

SERVES: 8

TIME: 35 minutes

Vegetable oil cooking spray
2 cups old-fashioned oats
1 teaspoon pumpkin pie spice
1 teaspoon baking soda

½ teaspoon ground cinnamon

½ cup maple syrup

1 (15-ounce) can pumpkin puree

2 eggs

Preheat the oven to 350°F. Spray a standard loaf pan with vegetable oil cooking spray.

In a large bowl, combine the oats, pumpkin pie spice, baking soda, and cinnamon. In a separate bowl, whisk together the maple syrup, pumpkin puree, and eggs. Pour the wet ingredients in with the dry ingredients. Mix well until combined. Use a hand mixer if the batter is thick.

Pour the batter into the prepared loaf pan. Bake for 30 to 35 minutes, until a toothpick pierced into the center comes out clean. Let cool for 10 minutes before slicing and serving.

No-Bake Cheesecake Bites

VF

SERVES: 8

TIME: 15 minutes, plus 1 hour in the freezer

Vegetable oil cooking spray

½ cup dates, pitted

½ cup almonds

1 teaspoon vanilla extract

¼ cup vegan cream cheese

6 tablespoons plain Greek yogurt (or almond yogurt if vegan)

1 tablespoon agave nectar

3 teaspoons stevia

2 teaspoons ground cinnamon

Spray 8 cups of a mini-muffin pan with the vegetable oil cooking spray.

In a food processor, blend the dates, almonds, vanilla, and 1 tablespoon of water until the mixture becomes sticky and dough-like. Press the mixture into each muffin cup to create the bottom of each mini cheese-cake. Clean the food processor bowl and blade.

In the food processor, blend the cream cheese, 4 tablespoons (¼ cup) of the Greek yogurt, the agave nectar, and 1 teaspoon of the stevia until well mixed. Evenly distribute this mixture on top of the base layer in the mini-muffin pan.

In a small bowl, mix the remaining 2 tablespoons of Greek yogurt, the cinnamon, and the remaining 2 teaspoons of stevia. Put a dollop on top of each mini cheesecake bite. Freeze until firm. Serve.

Tart Cherry Lime Gummies

SERVES: 12

TIME: 5 minutes, plus 1 hour in the refrigerator

1 cup organic tart cherry juice
Juice of 4 limes
⅛ cup beef gelatin powder
1 teaspoon honey

In a medium pot, combine the cherry juice, lime juice, gelatin powder, and honey. Cook over low heat for 5 minutes, stirring constantly. Use a candy dropper to put the liquid into molding trays and then refrigerate for at least 1 hour to set. Serve.

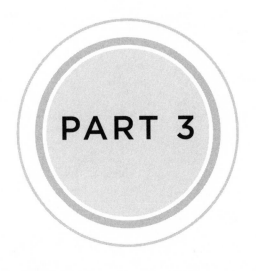

PART 3

POWER LIVING

8

POWER MOVES

Throughout this book, and in my daily life, I talk about the need for a lean and clean lifestyle. You can eat all the balanced meals, whole foods, and anti-inflammatory ingredients you want, but that's only part of the healthy equation—you must also exercise regularly. If you aren't physically active, all that hard work you put into your diet goes to waste (and maybe even your waist). A lack of regular exercise can put you on the fast track to weight gain and increase your risk of high blood pressure, heart disease, anxiety, and depression. A 2018 study found that a sedentary lifestyle is just as—if not more—detrimental to your health as smoking, high blood pressure, diabetes, cholesterol, and heart disease. By not exercising, you lose the power that a healthy, anti-inflammatory diet is trying to give your body. With my Power Moves, you're going to get that power back!

The Anti-Inflammatory Power of Exercise

I've really pounded out how important clean food is for fighting inflammation. Well, so is exercise. When you start exercising and moving your muscles, your muscle cells release small proteins that play a vital role in fighting inflammation, according to a review published in 2017 in the *European Journal of Clinical Investigation*. Basically, these special-forces proteins protect the body against substances that trigger inflammation. One of the proteins even keeps your body from putting on belly fat. How awesome is that for fat-proofing?

You can regulate how much of these proteins your muscles release—by the length of your workout. The longer you work out, the more of these anti-inflammatory proteins are released. But not to worry! All it takes is thirty minutes, and you increase these proteins by fivefold.

If there's ever a time to get moving, it's now. Stop making excuses and do it! You'll feel invigorated, lighter, and less stressed, and it will do your body a world of good.

Getting Started

As a general guideline, I recommend taking at least 10,000 steps per day. Try to take many of these steps outdoors—that way, you'll get a lot of natural health-protecting vitamin D from sunlight. Sun exposure is also great for boosting your immunity and your mood. Along with your steps, build in three or four days of weight training and cardio each week. For inspiration, my app Pretty Muscles provides thirty-minute workouts. The app is a terrific way to start improving your body, stamina, and overall health.

I firmly believe that working out can be fun—and that fun looks different for everyone. When you exercise, choose something you enjoy and it should never be an obligation or stress. That's why I've created my Power Games, which I describe in the next chapter. They make exercise a game, and games mean fun!

All of the Power Games involve plugging in various exercises that I call Power Moves, which I lay out in detail in this chapter. Since there are limitless combinations of Power Moves you can choose for each Power Game, you'll never get bored with exercise again!

THE POWER OF RESISTANCE BANDS

I rarely leave home without a set of resistance bands, whether they're to use myself or with one of my clients. They come in a variety of resistance levels (light, medium, heavy, etc.) and can be used virtually anywhere. Incorporating resistance bands into your workout can improve your muscle coordination, stability, and range of motion, and they're great for stretching your muscles— shoulders, back, chest, hamstrings, quads, glutes—before and after a workout. While I also sometimes use the loop-type bands (they look like thick rubber bands), the exercises here are to be done with the kind made of tubing and two handles.

Some Power Moves call for a resistance band that needs to be anchored in order to perform them correctly. Here are three convenient ways to go about it:

1. **Use a partner.** I often act as the resistance band anchor when training clients. If you have a workout buddy, take turns holding the band firmly as the other person performs the moves.
2. **Use a tree.** For a change of scenery, head outside and

(continued)

wrap the resistance band around the trunk of a sturdy tree.

3. **Use a door.** For this option, you'll need a sturdy door frame and an anchor strap attachment—it should have a loop at one end and an anchoring device (like a ring, or big foam plug) at the other. Place the strap between the door and the door frame, with the anchor end of the strap on the opposite side of the door from where you'll be exercising. Hold the loop end of the strap at the appropriate height, then close the door on the strap. Pull the strap until the anchor is snug against the other side of the door, then thread your resistance band through the loop end.

You'll adjust the position of the resistance band depending on the type of exercise. If you're using a partner, they'll simply hold it at the appropriate height, and if you're using a tree, you can shimmy the band up or down throughout your workout. If you're using a door, you can adjust the height of the strap by opening the door slightly and moving the anchor.

Power Moves

*Uses a resistance band

**Uses one or two weights

***Uses a jump rope

CORE AND BACK/LOWER BACK POWER MOVES

SKY DIVER: Lie on your stomach and stretch your arms behind you, as if you're diving headfirst out of a plane. Arch your back and lift your chest and legs as high as you can off the ground. Dip your chin in to relax your neck. Hold this position.

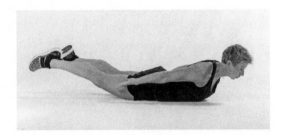

BICYCLE CRUNCH: Lie on your back with your hands by your ears, elbows wide. Bring your right elbow to your left knee, crunching as you meet in the middle. Your right leg remains extended and hovering just above the ground. Switch to your left elbow meeting your right knee, elbows remaining wide. Your left leg is extended and hovering just above the ground. Repeat at a controlled pace.

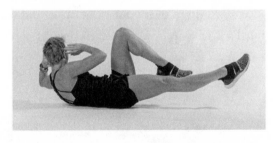

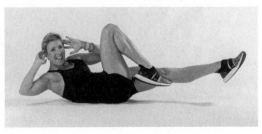

REGULAR CRUNCH: Lie on your back with your hands crossed over your chest or held lightly behind your head. Tilt your pelvis so your lower back is flat on the ground. Lift your chest up and use your abs to perform little pulses.

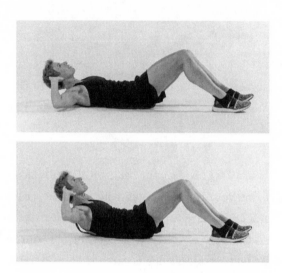

CRUNCH PULSES WITH LEGS STRAIGHT UP: Lie on your back with your hands crossed over your chest or behind your head and your legs extended straight up toward the ceiling. Crunch up and pulse toward your toes, never letting your shoulders hit the ground.

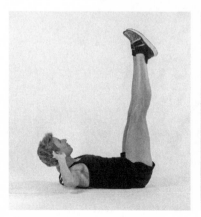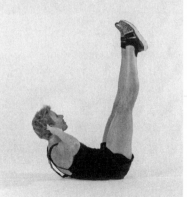

PLANK: Start on your hands and knees, with your hands underneath your shoulders. Engage your abs as you step both legs back to form a straight line from your feet to your head. Squeeze your booty and legs, making sure your back doesn't sag and your booty doesn't pop up toward the ceiling. Hold.

TIP: If a regular plank is too hard, drop to your knees, still keeping your core engaged.

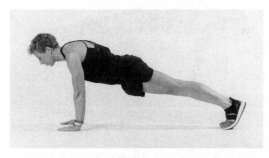

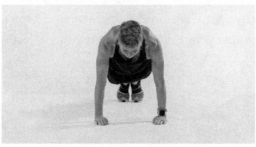

PLANK JACK: Get into the plank position. Jump your feet out wide and immediately jump back into the plank, like you're doing a jumping jack. Repeat.

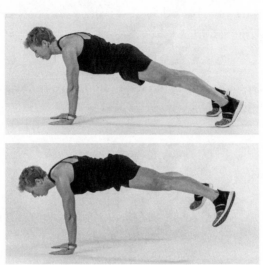

PLANK CHEST TAP: While holding the plank, bring one hand up at a time to tap your chest on the opposite side. Don't let your hips wiggle. The steadier your hips are the more it works your core! Repeat.

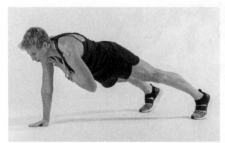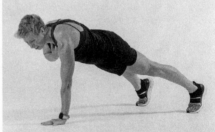

STRAIGHT LEG SIT-UP: Lie on your back with your legs extended flat on the ground. Raise your arms straight above your chest and sit straight up, never letting your legs lift. Slowly lower back to the starting position. That's one rep.

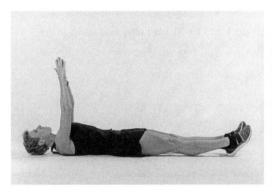
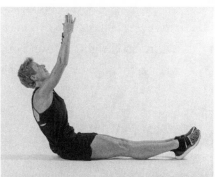

ELBOW PLANK WITH HIP DIP: Get into the plank position, resting on your elbows. Rotate your hips downward and dip them to the left side, then back up to the center. Then rotate your hips downward to the right, then back up to the center. Keep the rest of your body still the entire time. Think of it as making a rainbow with just your hips.

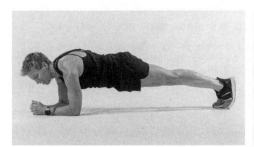
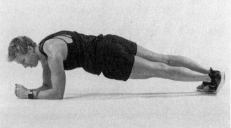

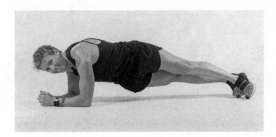

SIDE PLANK: Lie on your right side with your legs extended straight and feet stacked. Prop yourself up on your right forearm and hold your entire body tight, focusing on your abs and legs. Make sure your elbow is directly below your shoulder. Repeat on the other side.

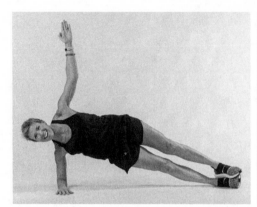 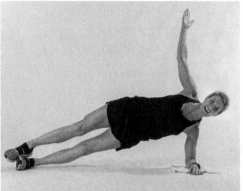

SIDE PLANK WITH HIP RAISE: Go into a side plank on your right forearm. Raise your left hip up to tuck in your right side (or oblique). Return to the starting position and continue to raise up and down. Think of this as little crunches for your sides! Repeat on the other side.

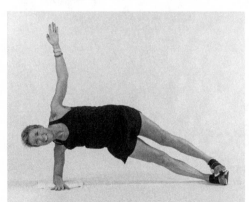 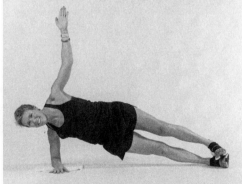

FLUTTER KICKS: Lie on your back with your legs extended straight and your hands underneath your booty to support your back. Lift your shoulders off the ground and engage your core. Now raise your legs about 6 inches off the ground and flutter your feet like you're kicking through water. Make sure to keep your legs stiff!

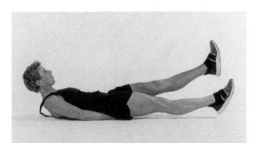 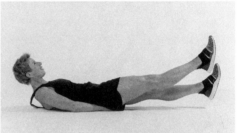

*BANDED ROW: Hold a band that's anchored in front of you, palms facing downward. Sit into a half squat to engage your legs. Pull your arms back, bringing your elbows tucked in to your sides, rotating your palms upward, and rotating your shoulders back to squeeze your shoulder blades behind you. That's one rep.

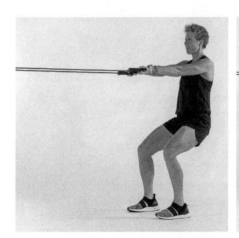 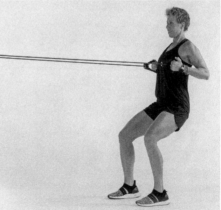

**BENT OVER ROW: Grab two weights (5 to 15 pounds) and go into a half squat with your hands hanging down, palms facing each other. Fall at the waist keeping your back flat and parallel to the ground throughout the entire maneuver. Now drive your elbows backward, keeping your elbows next to your body and NOT facing outward, squeezing your shoulder blades behind you. Release, return to the starting position, and repeat.

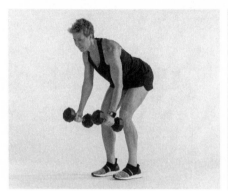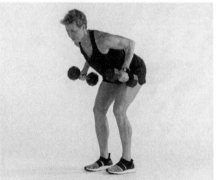

*ROW HOLD: Hold a band that's anchored in front of you, palms facing downward. Sit into a half squat to engage your legs. Pull your arms back, bringing your elbows tucked in to your sides, rotating your palms upward, and rotating your shoulders back to squeeze your shoulder blades behind you. Hold.

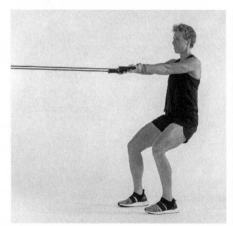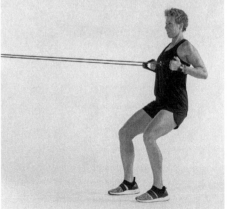

*SEATED WIDE PULL-DOWN: Anchor a band so it's above your head when you are seated. Sit down and grab the handles with your palms facing forward. Drive your elbows down and back, squeezing your shoulder blades together. Release and return to the starting position. That's one rep.

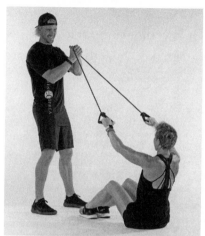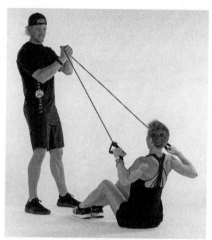

*SEATED WIDE PULL-DOWN HOLD: Anchor a band so it's above your head when you are seated. Sit down and grab the handles with your palms facing forward. Drive your elbows down and back, squeezing your shoulder blades together, and hold.

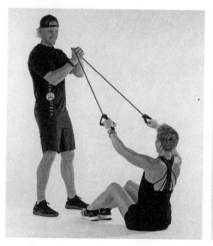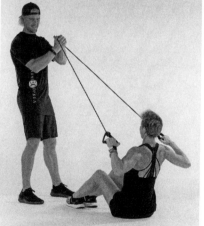

LEGS AND BOOTY POWER MOVES

REVERSE LUNGE: Stand with your weight on your left leg. Take a large step back with your right leg and drop your right knee straight down toward the ground until your left leg is parallel to the floor, never letting your right knee hit the floor. Driving through your left heel, return to the starting position with your right knee slightly lifted. That's one rep. Repeat on the other side.

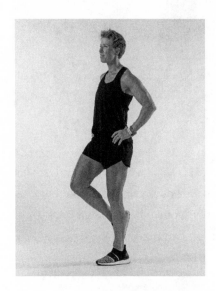

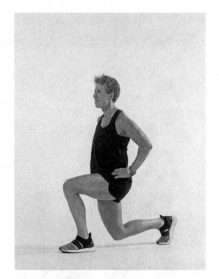

REVERSE LUNGE SWITCH: Go back into a lunge with your right leg and then come back to standing. Then switch legs and go back into a lunge with your left leg. Repeat this pattern, switching which leg goes back.

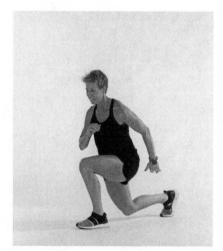
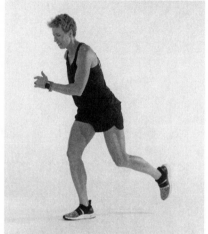
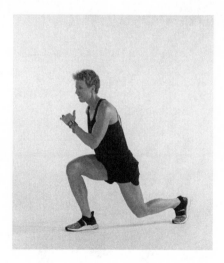

JUMPING LUNGE: Start in a left lunge position with your left leg at a 90-degree angle and your right knee straight down, hovering just above the floor. Now drive through your left heel and jump up, switching your foot placement in the air. Land softly. Repeat on the other side. That's one rep. Continue jumping and switching legs. Mega burner!

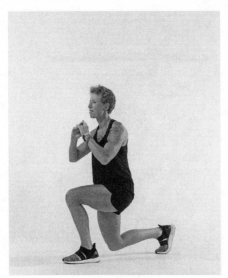
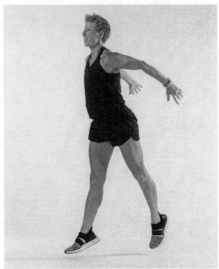

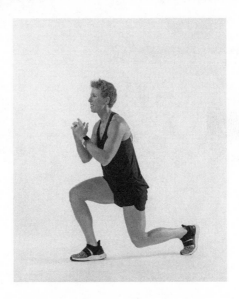

SUMO SQUAT: Stand with your legs out wide, toes at a 45-degree angle. Drop your booty until your legs are parallel to the ground, keeping your weight on your heels. Return to the starting position.

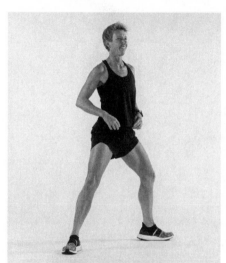 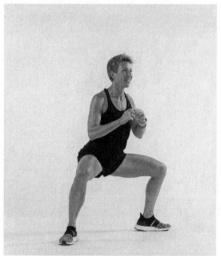

SUMO SQUAT PULSES: Put your feet out wide, toes turned out 45 degrees. Sink into a sumo squat and hold. Perform tiny pulses up and down.

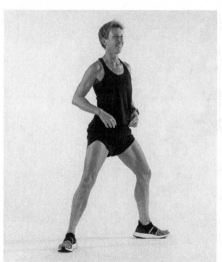 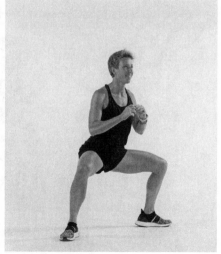

SUMO SQUAT JUMPS: Hold low in a sumo squat. Perform tiny jumps, staying low.

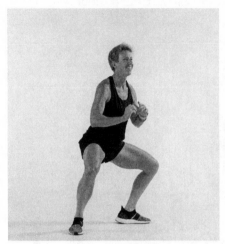
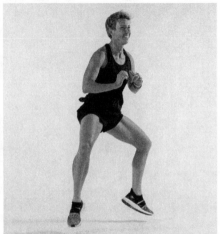

SUMO SQUAT HOLD: Perform a sumo squat and hold in a down position.

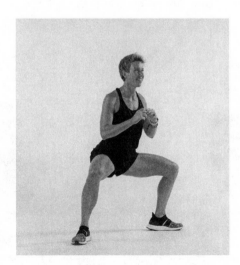

STATIONARY LUNGE: Take a big step back with your right leg and drop your right knee until it hovers just about the ground. Your left leg should be parallel to the ground. Keeping both feet in place, stand up. That's one rep.

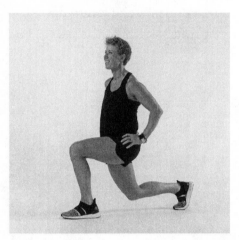

LUNGE HOLD: Perform a lunge and stay in the down position.

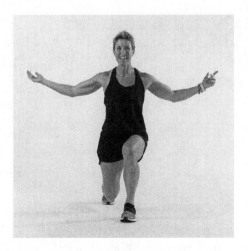

LUNGE PULSE WITH CHEST LEAN AND LEG LIFT: Start in a stationary lunge. Lean forward so that your chest is above your forward knee while continuing to hold your back flat. Drive through your front heel as you stand *halfway* up, lift your back leg slightly off the ground, squeeze your booty, and return down to repeat. The chest lean keeps your weight forward and increases the burn! Switch legs to get the other side.

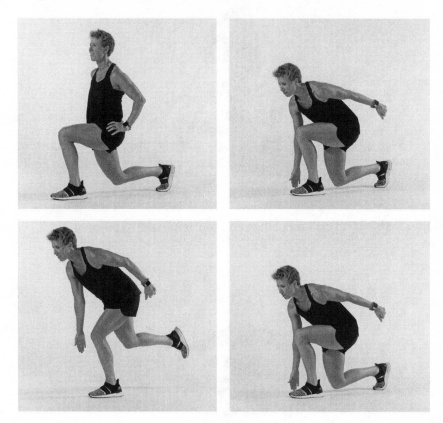

LATERAL LUNGE: Stand on your right leg, lunge to the left, and drop your booty until your left thigh is parallel to the ground. Keep your weight on your left heel and drive up to stand. Your right leg remains straight the entire time.

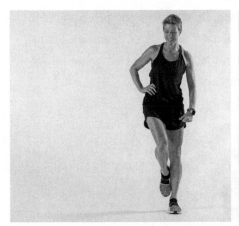
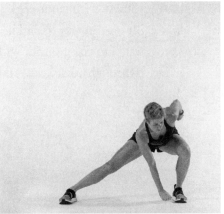

STATIONARY LATERAL LUNGE: Stand with your legs wider than hip-width apart. Perform a lateral lunge to the left without moving your feet. Drive through your left heel to immediately transition into a lateral lunge to the right. Push through your right heel now to return to the left. Continue lunging left and right, keeping your feet planted wide the entire time.

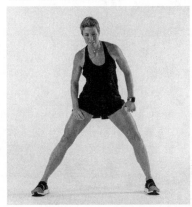
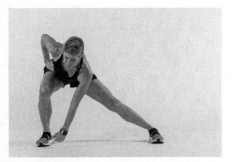
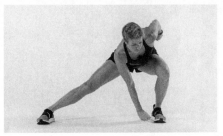

SQUAT: Stand with your legs shoulder-width apart, pelvis rotated back, weight on your heels, and head and chest up. Sit down until your legs are parallel to the ground, without letting your knees go past your toes. Drive through your heels, stand, and repeat.

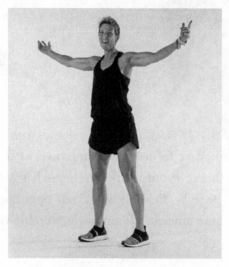

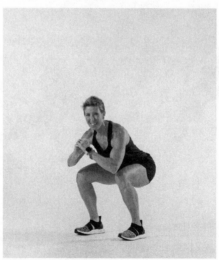

SQUAT JUMPS: Go down into a squat and from this low position drive up into the air, landing soft and straight back into a squat. Don't lock your legs as you land. Repeat!

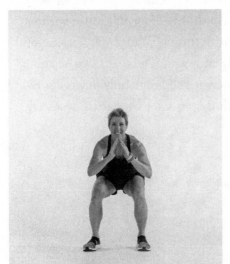 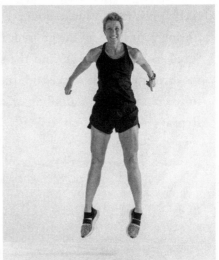

SQUAT HOLD: Perform a squat and hold in the down position, keeping your weight on your heels, shoulders back, and chest up.

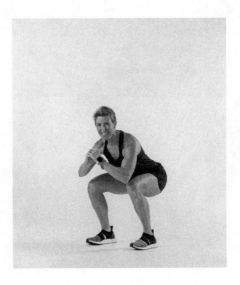

SQUAT INTO LUNGE: Stand with your legs shoulder-width apart, pelvis rotated back, weight on your heels, and head and chest up. Squat down on your left leg, while keeping your right toes lightly touching the floor for balance. Without fully standing up, move your right leg back so that you're in a lunge position. Go down into a full lunge without hitting your knee on the ground. Drive through your front heel as you stand halfway up to go into the squat again. These are two separate moves so make sure to get both the squat and lunge fully down but *not* fully up! Hold on to a railing or sturdy chair for support if necessary. Repeat.

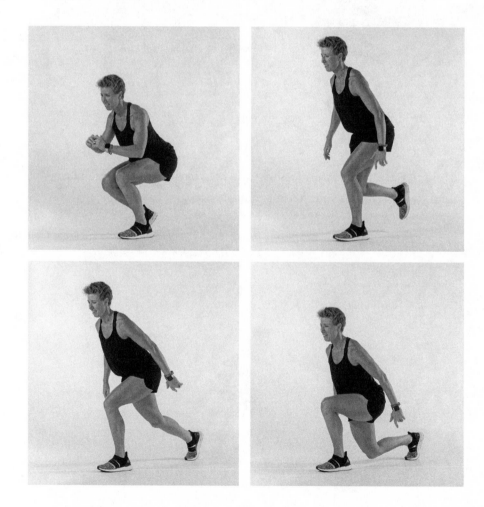

SQUAT SIDE KICK: Stand on your right leg, resting your left toes lightly on the floor for balance. Squat down so your right leg is parallel to the ground. Then, driving into your left heel, stand up halfway, kick your left leg out to the side. Return to the starting position without ever fully standing. Repeat on the other side.

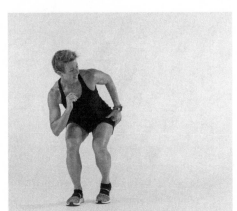
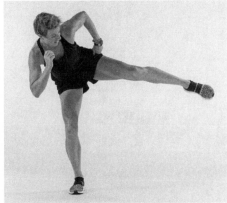

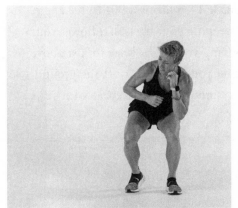
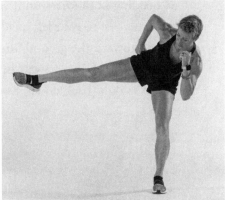

CURTSY LUNGE: Lunge back with your left leg and cross it behind your right leg, as if you were doing a curtsy. Bend both knees until your right leg forms a 90-degree angle. Keep your chest up. Return to the starting position, pushing through your right heel.

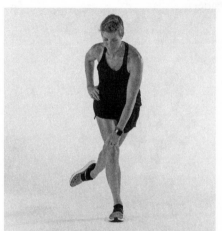 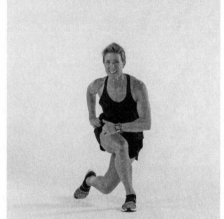

CURTSY LUNGE PULSE WITH CHEST LEAN: Perform a curtsy lunge, bending both knees until your left leg forms a 90-degree angle. Rotate your chest to your left quad, keeping your back flat. Lower your right hand toward the ground, dropping your right knee to just above the ground. Stand up partway, lifting your right foot off the ground, then drop it right back down, never standing fully. Repeat with your other leg.

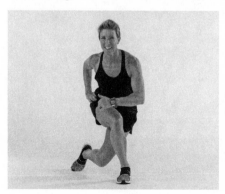 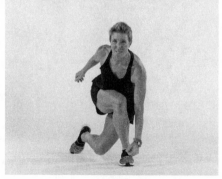

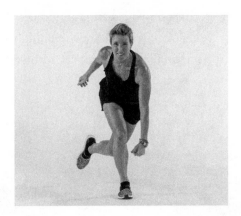

BRIDGE PULSES: Lie on your back, bend both legs, and put your weight on your heels. Bring your hips straight up in the air and push up and down, squeezing your booty and never letting your hips hit the ground.

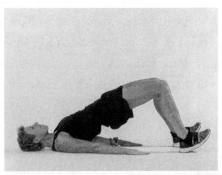

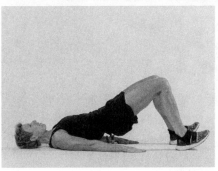

FIRE HYDRANT: Start on your hands and knees. Keeping your left knee bent, rotate your left hip until your left thigh is parallel to the floor. Return to the starting position. Repeat with your right leg.

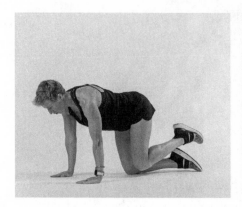
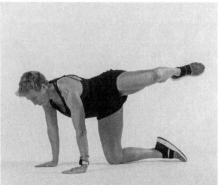

TABLE SLIDE: Start on your hands and knees and bring your left knee up into the high position of a fire hydrant. Now slide your left leg straight back until it is locked and fully extended, squeezing your booty tight and pointing your toes. Then slide your left knee back to the starting position, never letting your knee drop. Repeat with the other leg.

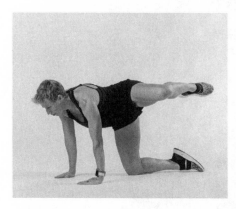
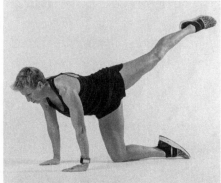

FIRE HYDRANT PULSES: Start on your hands and knees, and rotate your left hip until your left thigh is parallel to the floor, keeping your left knee bent. This is your starting position. Now lower your left knee halfway down and return to the starting position. Continue pulsing. Repeat with your right leg.

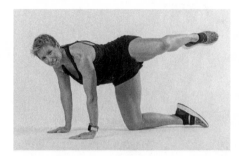 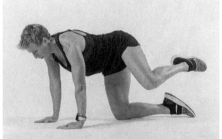

RAISED KNEE CIRCLES: Start on your hands and knees. Keeping your left knee bent, rotate your left hip until your left thigh is parallel to the floor. Rotate your left knee forward in tiny circles. Repeat with your other leg.

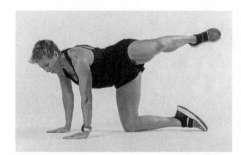 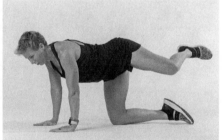

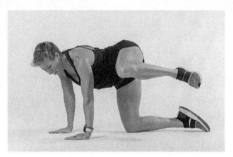

V BOOTY: Start on your hands and knees. Lock your left leg and lowering it on the other side of your right leg. Now bring your left leg directly upward, squeeze your booty, and lower it out to your left side, like you're drawing an upside-down V. Repeat with your right leg.

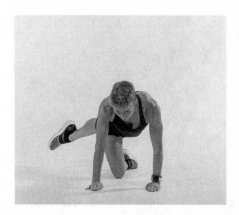
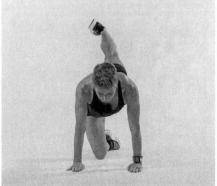

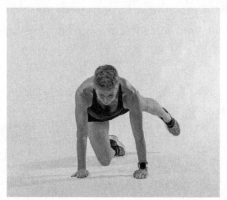

STRAIGHT LEG PULSES: Start on your hands and knees. Extend your left leg straight behind you, then make small pulses upward, squeezing your booty. Repeat with your right leg.

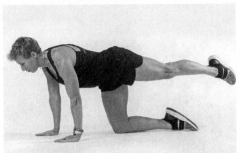 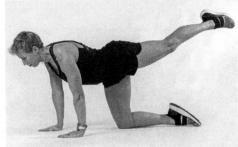

ARMS AND SHOULDERS POWER MOVES

FLOOR DIP: Sit on your booty with your knees bent, hands on the ground at your sides, and your fingers facing your feet. Push your hips off the ground into your starting position. Now bend your elbows, shooting them straight back. Push back up to the starting position. Repeat.

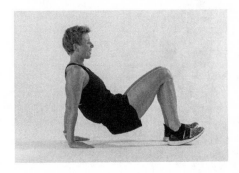 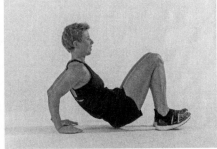

*BANDED BICEPS CURL: Anchor a resistance band low behind you. Step away from the anchor, then grab the handles with your palms facing up and pull your fists toward your shoulders. Keep your elbows glued to your sides. Return to the starting position. That's one rep.

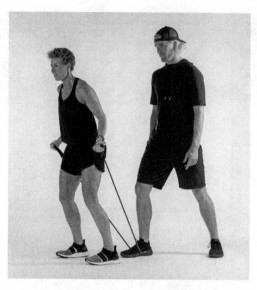

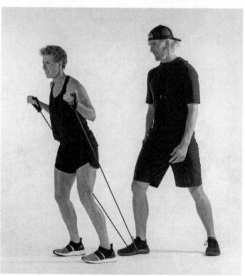

*BANDED BICEPS HOLD: Anchor a resistance band low behind you. Step away from the anchor, then grab the handles with your palms facing up and pull your fists toward your shoulders. Stop at 90 degrees, keeping your elbows glued to your sides, and hold.

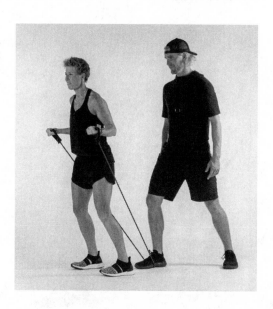

*BANDED TRICEPS EXTENSION: Anchor a resistance band in front of you, above your head. Use a door frame or high tree branch. Now grab the handles with your palms up and step back facing the anchor. Bend your arms to 90 degrees, then extend them down until your arms are squeezed straight. Return your elbows to 90 degrees and repeat.

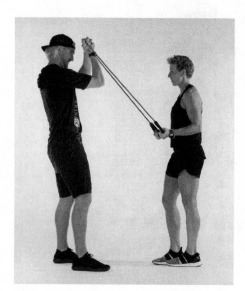 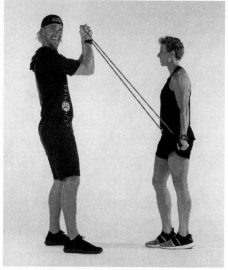

*BANDED TRICEPS PULSES: Anchor a resistance band in front of you, above your head. Use a door frame or high tree branch. Now grab the handles with your palms up, step back facing the anchor, and lock your arms at your sides. Now unlock your arms, then squeeze them straight again. (These are super-tiny bends in your elbow—then straighten your arms right back out.) Repeat. A movement as small as a pulse is hard to show in pictures and seeing my husband's corny smile makes me laugh, so you get this picture twice!

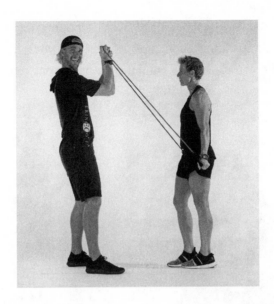

*BANDED REVERSE FLY: Anchor a resistance band in front of you, above your head. Grab the handles with your palms facing each other. Keeping a slight bend in your elbows, swing your arms out to your sides, squeezing your shoulder blades. Return your hands together in front of you. Repeat.

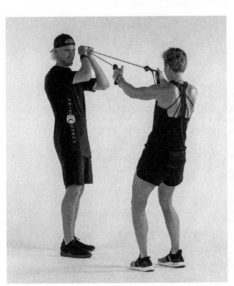 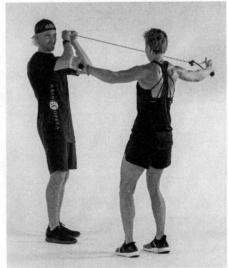

**BICEPS CURL: Grab a pair of 5- to 15-pound weights, turn your palms up, and curl the weights upward, keeping your elbows glued to your sides. Return to the starting position. That's one rep.

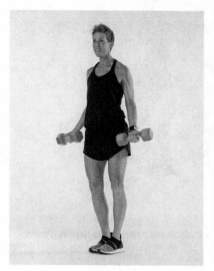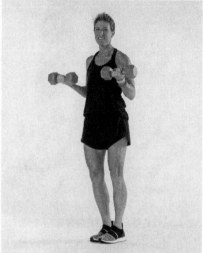

**BICEPS HOLD: Grab a pair of 5- to 15-pound weights, turn your palms up, curl the weights upward to 90 degrees, and hold.

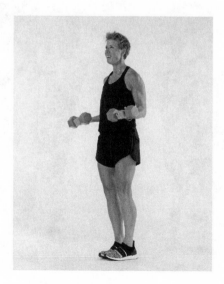

**HAMMER CURL: Grab a pair of 5- to 15-pound weights and grip them with your thumbs facing up, palms facing each other. Keeping your elbows glued to your sides, curl your arms up to your shoulders. Return to the starting position. That's one rep.

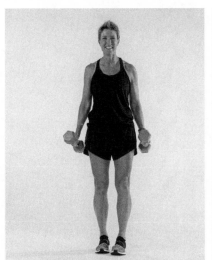 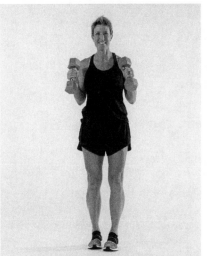

**TRICEPS KICKBACK: Grab a pair of 5- to 15-pound weights and fall forward at your waist, with your back flat and elbows bent 90 degrees at your sides. Extend both arms straight back, squeezing your triceps. Return to the starting position. That's one rep.

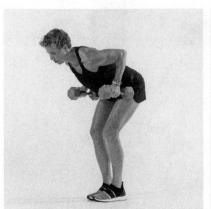 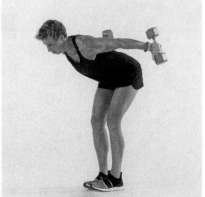

**OVERHEAD TRICEPS EXTENSION: Grab a 5- to 15-pound weight and hold it with both hands above your head, bending your elbows 90 degrees behind you. Then extend your arms straight up, squeezing your triceps as you straighten. Return to the starting position. That's one rep.

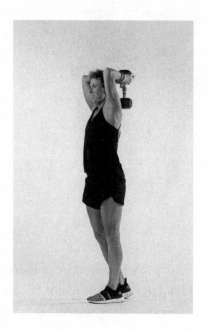

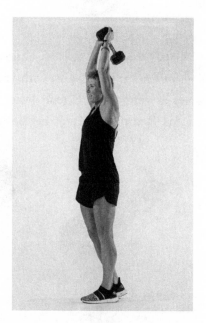

**W PULSES: Grab a pair of 3- to 8-pound weights and hold them out to the sides with your elbows bent and palms facing upward (forming a W). Bring your elbows slightly down to your ribs then back up and out, pulsing.

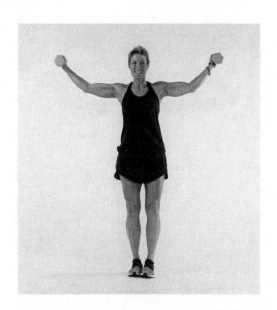

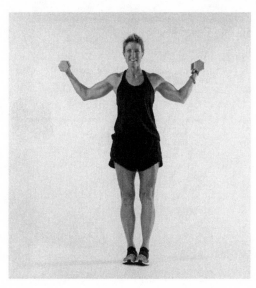

**LATERAL HOLD WITH BEND-IN: Grab a pair of 3- to 8-pound weights and hold them straight out to the sides with your palms facing down. Bend both elbows, leaving your arms at shoulder height and bring your hands into your chest. Keep your arms parallel to the ground the whole time. Repeat.

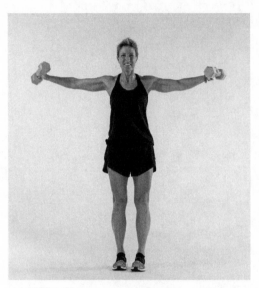

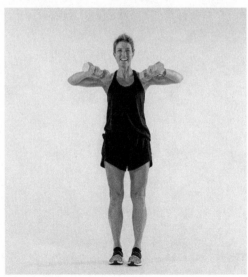

**LATERAL RAISE: Grab a pair of 3- to 15-pound weights and stand with your arms at your sides. Bend your elbows slightly, and keep your knees soft. Raise your arms straight out to the sides, up to shoulder level, elbows still soft. Return to the starting position. Repeat.

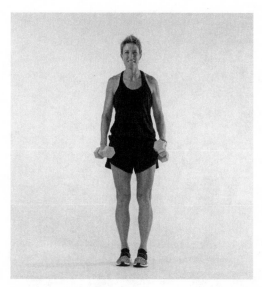

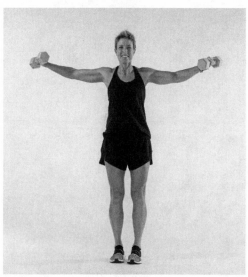

**FRONT V RAISE: Grab a pair of 3- to 15-pound weights and stand with your arms at your sides. Extend your locked arms in front of you up to shoulder level, creating a V in the air and keeping the weights vertical. Reverse in a controlled manner to return to the starting position. That's one rep.

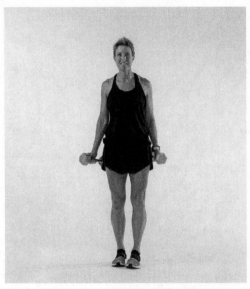

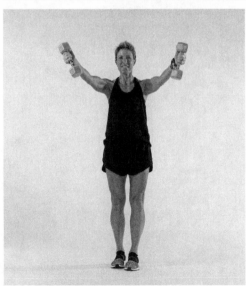

**SHOULDER PRESS: Grab a 3- to 20-pound weight in each hand. Hold the weights by your shoulders with your palms facing forward and your elbows out to the sides and bent at 90 degrees. Press the weights straight up until your arms are extended. Lower your arms back to 90 degrees. That's one rep.

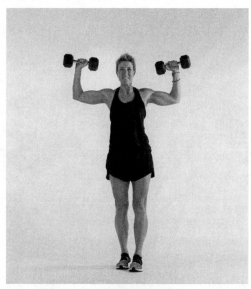

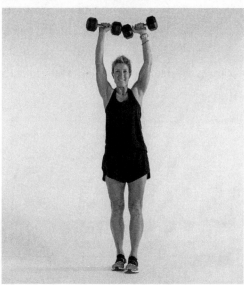

CHEST POWER MOVES

PUSH-UP: Get into the plank position, with your hands slightly wider than your shoulders. Lower your body toward the floor until your elbows are at 90 degrees. Push back to the starting position. That's one rep.

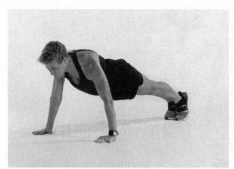 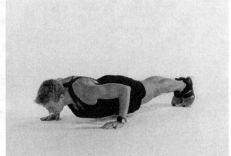

MILITARY PUSH-UP: Get into the plank position, placing your hands below your shoulders with your back and abs engaged. Bend your arms, elbows going straight back against your ribs, and lower your body until your elbows form 90 degrees and then push up from this position. That's one rep.

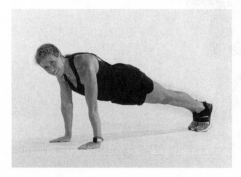 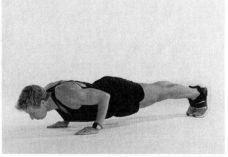

*BANDED CHEST PRESS: While standing, anchor a resistance band behind you at about shoulder level. Step one foot forward and lean forward slightly. Raise both arms so your shoulders and elbows are parallel with the ground. Push both arms forward until fully extended. Bring elbows back to even with your shoulders. That's one rep.

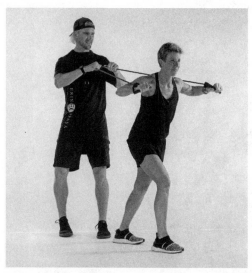

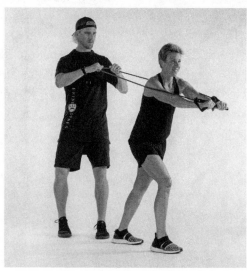

*BANDED CHEST FLY: While standing, anchor a resistance band behind you at about shoulder level. Step one foot forward and lean forward slightly. Raise both arms out to your sides so your shoulders and elbows are parallel with the ground. Keep a slight bend in your elbows, palms facing forward. While keeping your arms straight, bring your hands together in front of you, squeezing your chest in the process, and lightly touching your palms. Return your arms to the starting position. That's one rep.

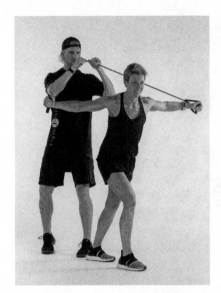

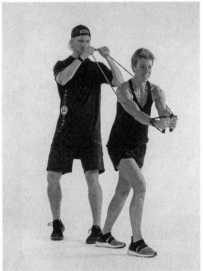

**CHEST PRESS: Grab two 10- to 25-pound weights, lie on your back, push your hips up into a bridge, and dig your heels into the ground. Put your arms out to the side, elbows hovering slightly above the ground. Press the weights straight up so your arms are fully extended. Return your arms to the starting position. That's one rep.

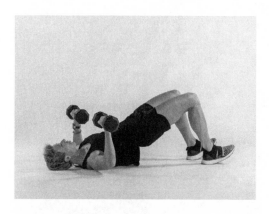

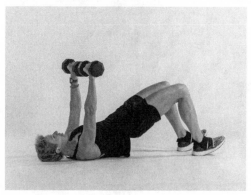

CARDIO POWER MOVES

JUMPING JACKS: Stand upright with your feet together and your arms by your sides. Jump and land with your feet shoulder-width apart, simultaneously raising your arms overhead. Jump back to the starting position and repeat.

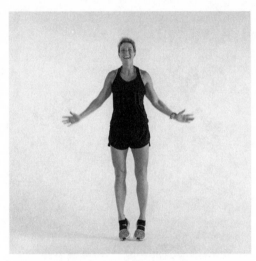

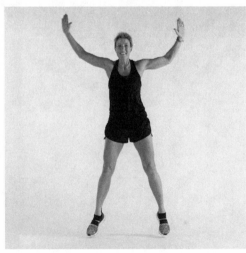

PLANK FROG JUMP: Get into the plank position. Keeping your hands on the ground, jump your legs forward so both feet land in a low sumo squat to the sides of your hands. Immediately jump back into the plank position, hands never leaving the ground and keeping your booty low the entire move. That's one rep.

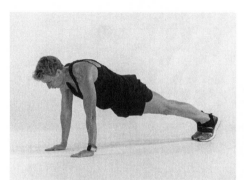 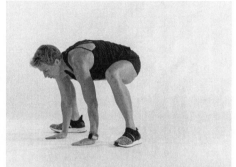

HIGH KNEES: Run in place, bringing each knee up in front of your body and keeping your core tight.

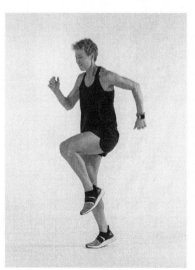 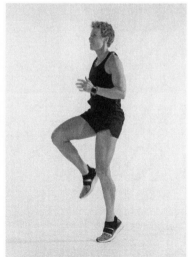

SKATER HOPS: Squat down on your right leg with your left leg bent behind you. Hop to the left, landing low on your left leg with your right leg swinging behind. Then hop back to the starting position and continue this motion like you're skating.

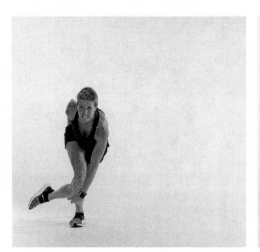

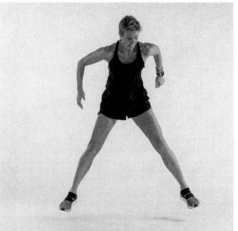

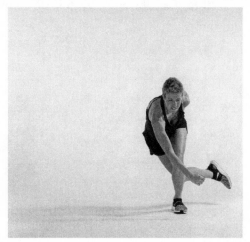

MOUNTAIN CLIMBERS: Get into the plank position. Drive your knees toward your chest one at a time, keeping your booty low and core tight. You should feel like you're running in place.

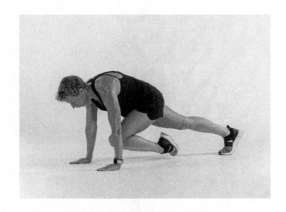

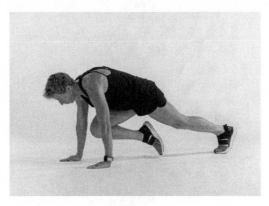

***JUMP ROPE:** Swing your arms and jump over the rope, keeping your arms bent and elbows close to your body. Repeat.

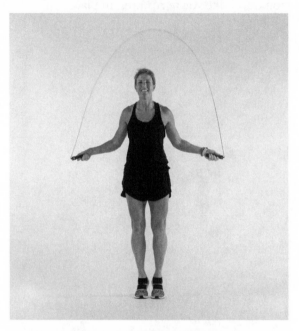

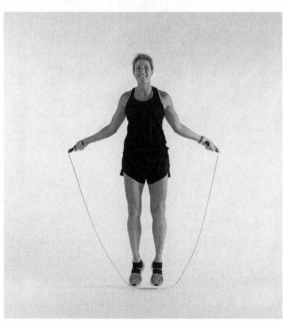

Power Moves galore! The essence of my workouts, just like my meal plan, is simplicity. You don't need to do fancy one-handed burpees to make Pretty Muscles! These are fantastic moves you should learn to master. What I suggest is that you get the hang of these moves by following the instructions and trying them out. Note which are your favorites. Apply your favorites to my Power Games, and you're on your way to a brand-new, super-fun way to work out.

9

POWER GAMES

The Power Games in this chapter work similarly to the Power
Plate meals. The "ingredients" of each game are the Power
Moves described in chapter 8, and you can use different combinations of them to create an unlimited number of workouts. For each
Power Game, I'll show you how to play it, how to play it with a partner,
and how to modify it for your fitness level. And to get you started, I'll
tell you the Power Move combinations that I regularly do with my clients. Try my examples or create your own combinations!

And remember to find your fun. My all-time favorite workout is
Tabata, and my husband takes his workouts outside whenever
possible—he likes anchoring a resistance band to playground equipment, for example. One of my clients frequently requests the Reverse
Pyramid game (see page 270), while another loves to turn Hit the Deck
(see page 277) into a friendly competition with her husband. Start by
swapping out one of your regular workouts for a Power Game, then try
another one, and see which ones you look forward to doing again and

again. I hope one of these games becomes *your* new favorite way to work out.

PREP YOUR BODY

To prevent injury and increase your flexibility, make sure you warm up before each workout and cool down afterward.

HOW TO POWER UP
Dedicate five minutes to warming up before each workout. A brisk walk, jumping rope, or jumping jacks followed by leg swings (front and back, then side to side) are my go-tos.

HOW TO POWER DOWN
To lower your heart rate after all that hard work, cool down by walking for a couple of minutes and then holding several stretches—targeting your quads, hamstrings, glutes, chest, and shoulders—for ten to thirty seconds each. I also love using a foam roller to relieve any tension.

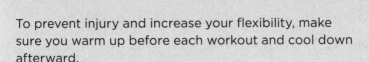

Power Game #1: Classic Tabata

For me, it doesn't get more fun than the Tabata—it's a high-intensity workout that lasts only four minutes. This form of exercise has completely changed the way I work out and the results I see, which in turn has completely changed the way my clients work out and the results they see.

A Tabata is a twenty-second burst of exercise, followed by ten seconds of rest, for eight rounds. Altogether, that's four minutes. You can do the same exercise eight times or alternate rounds; either way, by the time you're done, you should be *beat*. It might be easier to understand when written out like this:

Round #1: 20 seconds of all-out exercise; 10 seconds of rest

Round #2: 20 seconds of all-out exercise; 10 seconds of rest

Round #3: 20 seconds of all-out exercise; 10 seconds of rest

Round #4: 20 seconds of all-out exercise; 10 seconds of rest

Round #5: 20 seconds of all-out exercise; 10 seconds of rest

Round #6: 20 seconds of all-out exercise; 10 seconds of rest

Round #7: 20 seconds of all-out exercise; 10 seconds of rest

Round #8: 20 seconds of all-out exercise; 10 seconds of rest

I discovered Tabata several years ago while reading about its effectiveness in a fitness article. I did some extra digging and learned that Tabata got its big break in the 1990s thanks to a health-science researcher and speed-skating coach named Dr. Izumi Tabata. He led a study that had one group of male college students ride a stationary bike at moderate intensity for one hour, five days a week, and a second group of male college students perform a stationary bike Tabata—which is twenty seconds of pedaling possibly the hardest they've ever pedaled, then ten seconds of rest, repeated eight times—four times a week.

Over six weeks, Dr. Tabata and his team studied each participant's anaerobic capacity (how long he or she could perform an exercise with maximum exertion) and VO_2 max (the highest amount of oxygen his or her body could transport and use for energy during exercise); at its core, they were comparing a one-hour workout with a four-minute workout. The results, published in a 1996 issue of *Medicine and Science in Sports and Exercise*, were shocking: Variables notwithstanding, four minutes of super-high-intensity cycling was significantly more effective than an hour of moderate cycling. Incredible!

I took that idea and ran with it, using the Tabata format for all the exercises I'd already been doing: squats, push-ups, sit-ups, mountain climbers, all kinds of weighted and non-weighted arm exercises, even plain old sprints. I found that it works for pretty much any basic workout move you can think of. Actually, it's best when paired with simple exercises! The only equipment you need is a Tabata timer, which you can download on your smartphone or find on my app, Pretty Muscles.

Dr. Tabata's study showed that his four-minute workouts can dramatically improve your VO_2 max, which is an important indicator of your heart and lung health. The higher your VO_2 max, the more oxygen your body can use and deliver to your muscles.

Tabata has tons of other benefits, too: It can be done anywhere, anytime—try it in your kitchen, driveway, or hallway. I've found that Tabata forces you to challenge yourself, because you only have twenty seconds of intense movement at a time.

TABATA TIPS AND TRICKS

If you've never done a Tabata before, you're about to enter a whole new world of exercise. Here are a few words of wisdom to keep in mind before diving into the Tabata combinations in this chapter.

1. Start with your favorite Power Moves as you're mastering the format—it's easy once you get the hang of it, but your first Tabata might take a few tries. For a simple lower-body blast, try alternating rounds of reverse lunge switch and squat jumps.
2. Pretend it's a game—because games are, by default, fun! To really make it a workout party, put on some upbeat music. (I have a Spotify and Apple Music playlist called "Erin Oprea Workout Party," if you need inspiration.)

(continued)

3. If you're struggling to get through the eight bursts of exercise, remind yourself that you can do anything for twenty seconds. Anything!
4. When your muscles start to burn, go to a happy place mentally—like a spa, beach, or early 2000 rap—and keep pushing through the pain.
5. Above all else, make sure you're using good form, because this is how you get the most out of any workout. Turn to pages 208–56 to see seventy of the best moves for Tabata and how to do them properly.
6. With Power Moves that don't require equipment like a resistance band or weights, you can do Tabata anywhere.

HOW TO PLAY

STEP 1: Learn the Tabata format:

- A Tabata is a four-minute workout that consists of eight rounds.
- Each round consists of twenty-second bursts of exercise followed by ten seconds of rest.
- Each twenty-second burst of exercise should be an all-out effort.

STEP 2: Use a Tabata app or download my app, Pretty Muscles, to use as your timer—this is the easiest way to count out each round. Get familiar with using the app before diving into the actual exercises.

STEP 3: Pick two Power Moves to perform, keeping in mind that you'll do four rounds of each one. You'll use this format:

POWER MOVE #1 + POWER MOVE #2

Round 1: Power Move #1 for 20 seconds, rest for 10 seconds

Round 2: Power Move #2 for 20 seconds, rest for 10 seconds

Round 3: Power Move #1 for 20 seconds, rest for 10 seconds

Round 4: Power Move #2 for 20 seconds, rest for 10 seconds

Round 5: Power Move #1 for 20 seconds, rest for 10 seconds

Round 6: Power Move #2 for 20 seconds, rest for 10 seconds

Round 7: Power Move #1 for 20 seconds, rest for 10 seconds

Round 8: Power Move #2 for 20 seconds, rest for 10 seconds

HOW TO PLAY WITH A PARTNER

With a partner Tabata workout, there are still eight rounds of two different Power Moves. In Round 1, you perform Power Move #1, and your partner performs Power Move #2. In Round 2, you switch. Continue to trade off until you complete all eight rounds.

HOW TO MODIFY FOR YOUR FITNESS LEVEL

All of the Tabata combinations that follow are at an intermediate fitness level, so try these if you are already physically active. Below each Tabata are ways to make it both easier (modify down) and harder (modify up).

MY FAVORITE POWER MOVE COMBINATIONS

#1: SKY DIVERS + BICYCLE CRUNCHES

Round 1: Sky divers for 20 seconds, rest for 10 seconds

Round 2: Bicycle crunches for 20 seconds, rest for 10 seconds

Round 3: Sky divers for 20 seconds, rest for 10 seconds

Round 4: Bicycle crunches for 20 seconds, rest for 10 seconds

Round 5: Sky divers for 20 seconds, rest for 10 seconds

Round 6: Bicycle crunches for 20 seconds, rest for 10 seconds

Round 7: Sky divers for 20 seconds, rest for 10 seconds

Round 8: Bicycle crunches for 20 seconds, rest for 10 seconds

MODIFY DOWN
Sky divers + regular crunches

MODIFY UP
8 rounds of sky divers + 8 rounds of bicycle crunches (2 Tabata! Get it?)

#2: JUMPING LUNGES + SUMO SQUAT JUMPS

Round 1: Jumping lunges for 20 seconds, rest for 10 seconds

Round 2: Sumo squat jumps for 20 seconds, rest for 10 seconds

Round 3: Jumping lunges for 20 seconds, rest for 10 seconds

Round 4: Sumo squat jumps for 20 seconds, rest for 10 seconds

Round 5: Jumping lunges for 20 seconds, rest for 10 seconds

Round 6: Sumo squat jumps for 20 seconds, rest for 10 seconds

Round 7: Jumping lunges for 20 seconds, rest for 10 seconds

Round 8: Sumo squat jumps for 20 seconds, rest for 10 seconds

MODIFY DOWN
Reverse lunge switches + sumo squats

MODIFY UP
8 rounds of jumping lunges + 8 rounds of sumo squat jumps

#3: CURTSY LUNGE PULSES WITH CHEST LEAN ON LEFT LEG + CURTSY LUNGE PULSES WITH CHEST LEAN ON RIGHT LEG

Round 1: Curtsy lunge pulses with chest lean on left leg for 20 seconds, rest for 10 seconds

Round 2: Curtsy lunge pulses with chest lean on right leg for 20 seconds, rest for 10 seconds

Round 3: Curtsy lunge pulses with chest lean on left leg for 20 seconds, rest for 10 seconds

Round 4: Curtsy lunge pulses with chest lean on right leg for 20 seconds, rest for 10 seconds

Round 5: Curtsy lunge pulses with chest lean on left leg for 20 seconds, rest for 10 seconds

Round 6: Curtsy lunge pulses with chest lean on right leg for 20 seconds, rest for 10 seconds

Round 7: Curtsy lunge pulses with chest lean on left leg for 20 seconds, rest for 10 seconds

Round 8: Curtsy lunge pulses with chest lean on right leg for 20 seconds, rest for 10 seconds

MODIFY DOWN
Curtsy lunge pulses on left leg with chest up + curtsy lunge pulses on right leg with chest up

MODIFY UP
- 8 rounds of curtsy lunge pulses with chest lean on left leg + 8 rounds of curtsy lunge pulses with chest lean on right leg
- Add weights.

#4: V BOOTY LEFT + V BOOTY RIGHT

Round 1: V booty left for 20 seconds, rest for 10 seconds

Round 2: V booty right for 20 seconds, rest for 10 seconds

Round 3: V booty left for 20 seconds, rest for 10 seconds

Round 4: V booty right for 20 seconds, rest for 10 seconds

Round 5: V booty left for 20 seconds, rest for 10 seconds

Round 6: V booty right for 20 seconds, rest for 10 seconds

Round 7: V booty left for 20 seconds, rest for 10 seconds

Round 8: V booty right for 20 seconds, rest for 10 seconds

MODIFY DOWN
Straight leg pulses right + straight leg pulses left

MODIFY UP
8 rounds of V booty left + 8 rounds of V booty right

#5: BICEPS CURLS + HAMMER CURLS

Round 1: Biceps curls for 20 seconds, rest for 10 seconds

Round 2: Hammer curls for 20 seconds, rest for 10 seconds

Round 3: Biceps curls for 20 seconds, rest for 10 seconds

Round 4: Hammer curls for 20 seconds, rest for 10 seconds

Round 5: Biceps curls for 20 seconds, rest for 10 seconds

Round 6: Hammer curls for 20 seconds, rest for 10 seconds

Round 7: Biceps curls for 20 seconds, rest for 10 seconds

Round 8: Hammer curls for 20 seconds, rest for 10 seconds

Use lighter weights for all 8 rounds.

Use heavier weights for all 8 rounds.

#6: CHEST PRESSES + OVERHEAD TRICEPS EXTENSIONS

Round 1: Chest presses for 20 seconds, rest for 10 seconds

Round 2: Overhead triceps extensions for 20 seconds, rest for 10 seconds

Round 3: Chest presses for 20 seconds, rest for 10 seconds

Round 4: Overhead triceps extensions for 20 seconds, rest for 10 seconds

Round 5: Chest presses for 20 seconds, rest for 10 seconds

Round 6: Overhead triceps extensions for 20 seconds, rest for 10 seconds

Round 7: Chest presses for 20 seconds, rest for 10 seconds

Round 8: Overhead triceps extensions for 20 seconds, rest for 10 seconds

MODIFY DOWN
Use lighter weights for all 8 rounds.

MODIFY UP
Use heavier weights for all 8 rounds.

#7: PLANK CHEST TAPS + PLANK

Round 1: Plank chest taps for 20 seconds, rest for 10 seconds

Round 2: Plank for 20 seconds, rest for 10 seconds

Round 3: Plank chest taps for 20 seconds, rest for 10 seconds

Round 4: Plank for 20 seconds, rest for 10 seconds

Round 5: Plank chest taps for 20 seconds, rest for 10 seconds

Round 6: Plank for 20 seconds, rest for 10 seconds

Round 7: Plank chest taps for 20 seconds, rest for 10 seconds

Round 8: Plank for 20 seconds, rest for 10 seconds

MODIFY DOWN
Plank on your knees + plank

MODIFY UP
8 rounds of plank chest taps

#8: STATIONARY LUNGES WITH LEFT LEG IN FRONT + STATIONARY LUNGES RIGHT/RIGHT LEG IN FRONT

Round 1: Stationary lunges with left leg in front for 20 seconds, rest for 10 seconds

Round 2: Stationary lunges with right leg in front for 20 seconds, rest for 10 seconds

Round 3: Stationary lunges with left leg in front for 20 seconds, rest for 10 seconds

Round 4: Stationary lunges with right leg in front for 20 seconds, rest for 10 seconds

Round 5: Stationary lunges with left leg in front for 20 seconds, rest for 10 seconds

Round 6: Stationary lunges with right leg in front for 20 seconds, rest for 10 seconds

Round 7: Stationary lunges with left leg in front for 20 seconds, rest for 10 seconds

Round 8: Stationary lunges with right leg in front for 20 seconds, rest for 10 seconds

MODIFY DOWN
Hold on to a wall for stability for all 8 rounds.

MODIFY UP
Add weights for all 8 rounds.

#9: LATERAL LUNGES ON LEFT + LATERAL LUNGES ON RIGHT

Round 1: Lateral lunges on left for 20 seconds, rest for 10 seconds

Round 2: Lateral lunges on right for 20 seconds, rest for 10 seconds

Round 3: Lateral lunges on left for 20 seconds, rest for 10 seconds

Round 4: Lateral lunges on right for 20 seconds, rest for 10 seconds

Round 5: Lateral lunges on left for 20 seconds, rest for 10 seconds

Round 6: Lateral lunges on right for 20 seconds, rest for 10 seconds

Round 7: Lateral lunges on left for 20 seconds, rest for 10 seconds

Round 8: Lateral lunges on right for 20 seconds, rest for 10 seconds

MODIFY DOWN
Stationary lateral lunges on left + stationary lateral lunges on right

MODIFY UP
- 8 rounds of lateral lunges on left, 8 rounds of lateral lunge on right
- Add weights.

#10: SQUATS + SQUAT HOLDS

Round 1: Squats for 20 seconds, rest for 10 seconds

Round 2: Squat holds for 20 seconds, rest for 10 seconds

Round 3: Squats for 20 seconds, rest for 10 seconds

Round 4: Squat holds for 20 seconds, rest for 10 seconds

Round 5: Squats for 20 seconds, rest for 10 seconds

Round 6: Squat holds for 20 seconds, rest for 10 seconds

Round 7: Squats for 20 seconds, rest for 10 seconds

Round 8: Squat holds for 20 seconds, rest for 10 seconds

MODIFY DOWN
Hold on to a wall for stability for all 8 rounds.

MODIFY UP
- 8 rounds of squat jumps
- Add weights.

Power Game #2: Reverse Pyramid

This is a mind game as much as it is a Power Game! Because you're doing a fewer number of reps in each round, your brain will think things get easier as you near the finish line. But your body is actually working harder because you've front-loaded all of your effort.

HOW TO PLAY
Pick two Power Moves to use throughout the game. Start by doing ten of the first move, then ten of the second move. Then immediately do nine of the first move, then nine of the second move. Then immediately do eight of the first move, then eight of the second move. Continue this pattern all the way down to one, without stopping. If you choose a Power Move that involves a hold (like a plank), a pulse (like a sumo squat pulse), or cardio (like jumping jacks), perform for ten seconds rather than doing the corresponding number of reps.

HOW TO PLAY WITH A PARTNER

You and a partner can do the same moves at the same time, round for round, pushing each other to keep up. Or, if you only have one pair of weights or one resistance band, you can alternate the moves every round—you do Power Move #1 while your partner does Power Move #2, then switch.

You'll use this format:

10 Power Move #1 + 10 Power Move #2

9 Power Move #1 + 9 Power Move #2

8 Power Move #1 + 8 Power Move #2

7 Power Move #1 + 7 Power Move #2

6 Power Move #1 + 6 Power Move #2

5 Power Move #1 + 5 Power Move #2

4 Power Move #1 + 4 Power Move #2

3 Power Move #1 + 3 Power Move #2

2 Power Move #1 + 2 Power Move #2

1 Power Move #1 + 1 Power Move #2

HOW TO MODIFY FOR YOUR FITNESS LEVEL

MODIFY DOWN

- Start your countdown at 5 rather than 10. Next time, start at 6 and work up to starting at 10.
- Start your countdown at 10 but only do the even-numbered rounds: 10, 8, 6, 4, 2.

MODIFY UP

Choose Power Moves that use weights, like biceps curls or chest presses, and increase the amount of weight once it becomes easy.

MY FAVORITE POWER MOVE COMBINATIONS

#1: SHOULDER PRESSES ON KNEES + PUSH-UPS

10 shoulder presses on knees + 10 push-ups

9 shoulder presses on knees + 9 push-ups

8 shoulder presses on knees + 8 push-ups

7 shoulder presses on knees + 7 push-ups

6 shoulder presses on knees + 6 push-ups

5 shoulder presses on knees + 5 push-ups

4 shoulder presses on knees + 4 push-ups

3 shoulder presses on knees + 3 push-ups

2 shoulder presses on knees + 2 push-ups

1 shoulder press on knees + 1 push-up

#2: SQUAT SIDE KICKS LEFT + SQUAT SIDE KICKS RIGHT

10 squat side kicks left + 10 squat side kicks right

9 squat side kicks left + 9 squat side kicks right

8 squat side kicks left + 8 squat side kicks right

7 squat side kicks left + 7 squat side kicks right

6 squat side kicks left + 6 squat side kicks right

5 squat side kicks left + 5 squat side kicks right

4 squat side kicks left + 4 squat side kicks right

3 squat side kicks left + 3 squat side kicks right

2 squat side kicks left + 2 squat side kicks right

1 squat side kick left + 1 squat side kick right

#3: LATERAL RAISES + TRICEPS KICKBACKS

10 lateral raises + 10 triceps kickbacks

9 lateral raises + 9 triceps kickbacks

8 lateral raises + 8 triceps kickbacks

7 lateral raises + 7 triceps kickbacks

6 lateral raises + 6 triceps kickbacks

5 lateral raises + 5 triceps kickbacks

4 lateral raises + 4 triceps kickbacks

3 lateral raises + 3 triceps kickbacks

2 lateral raises + 2 triceps kickbacks

1 lateral raise + 1 triceps kickback

#4: FLOOR DIPS + OVERHEAD TRICEPS EXTENSIONS

10 floor dips + 10 overhead triceps extensions

9 floor dips + 9 overhead triceps extensions

8 floor dips + 8 overhead triceps extensions

7 floor dips + 7 overhead triceps extensions

6 floor dips + 6 overhead triceps extensions

5 floor dips + 5 overhead triceps extensions

4 floor dips + 4 overhead triceps extensions

3 floor dips + 3 overhead triceps extensions

2 floor dips + 2 overhead triceps extensions

1 floor dip + 1 overhead triceps extension

TIP: Perform the overhead triceps extensions on your knees, rather than standing, since you'll already be on the floor for the dips.

#5: BANDED ROWS + ROW HOLDS

10 banded rows + 10 seconds of row hold

9 banded rows + 10 seconds of row hold

8 banded rows + 10 seconds of row hold

7 banded rows + 10 seconds of row hold

6 banded rows + 10 seconds of row hold

5 banded rows + 10 seconds of row hold

4 banded rows + 10 seconds of row hold

3 banded rows + 10 seconds of row hold

2 banded rows + 10 seconds of row hold

1 banded row + 10 seconds of row hold

TIP: It's a good idea to time your 10 seconds, which is easily done by counting out loud. That way, you get the full benefit of the 10-second intervals and never shortchange yourself by doing less.

#6: BICEPS CURLS + BICEPS HOLDS

10 biceps curls + 10 seconds of biceps hold

9 biceps curls + 10 seconds of biceps hold

8 biceps curls + 10 seconds of biceps hold

7 biceps curls + 10 seconds of biceps hold

6 biceps curls + 10 seconds of biceps hold

5 biceps curls + 10 seconds of biceps hold

4 biceps curls + 10 seconds of biceps hold

3 biceps curls + 10 seconds of biceps hold

2 biceps curls + 10 seconds of biceps hold

1 biceps curl + 10 seconds of biceps hold

#7: SQUAT JUMPS + SQUAT HOLDS

10 squat jumps + 10 seconds of squat hold

9 squat jumps + 10 seconds of squat hold

8 squat jumps + 10 seconds of squat hold

7 squat jumps + 10 seconds of squat hold

6 squat jumps + 10 seconds of squat hold

5 squat jumps + 10 seconds of squat hold

4 squat jumps + 10 seconds of squat hold

3 squat jumps + 10 seconds of squat hold

2 squat jumps + 10 seconds of squat hold

1 squat jump + 10 seconds of squat hold

#8: PUSH-UPS + PLANK

10 push-ups + 10 seconds of plank

9 push-ups + 10 seconds of plank

8 push-ups + 10 seconds of plank

7 push-ups + 10 seconds of plank

6 push-ups + 10 seconds of plank

5 push-ups + 10 seconds of plank

4 push-ups + 10 seconds of plank

3 push-ups + 10 seconds of plank

2 push-ups + 10 seconds of plank

1 push-up + 10 seconds of plank

#9: SUMO SQUATS + SUMO SQUAT HOLDS

10 sumo squats + 10 seconds of sumo squat hold

9 sumo squats + 10 seconds of sumo squat hold

8 sumo squats + 10 seconds of sumo squat hold

7 sumo squats + 10 seconds of sumo squat hold

6 sumo squats + 10 seconds of sumo squat hold

5 sumo squats + 10 seconds of sumo squat hold

4 sumo squats + 10 seconds of sumo squat hold

3 sumo squats + 10 seconds of sumo squat hold

2 sumo squats + 10 seconds of sumo squat hold

1 sumo squat + 10 seconds of sumo squat hold

#10: SQUATS + SQUAT HOLDS

10 squats + 10 seconds of squat hold

9 squats + 10 seconds of squat hold

8 squats + 10 seconds of squat hold

7 squats + 10 seconds of squat hold

6 squats + 10 seconds of squat hold

5 squats + 10 seconds of squat hold

4 squats + 10 seconds of squat hold

3 squats + 10 seconds of squat hold

2 squats + 10 seconds of squat hold

1 squat + 10 seconds of squat hold

TIP: Notice a lot of squats in these Reverse Pyramid combinations? They're a staple of my training sessions and how many of my clients earn their toned legs!

Power Game #3: Hit the Deck

One of my clients inspired this game—which is a nice change from me telling them what to do all the time! Hit the Deck is a race to get through an entire deck of cards using four sets of Power Moves. Because you determine what those four moves are, it can be a completely new game every time you play it. I'm sure you have a deck of cards lying around your house—now put it to use! My app, Pretty Muscles, also has a digital version of Hit the Deck.

HOW TO PLAY

Grab a deck of cards and assign each of the four suits—clubs, diamonds, hearts, spades—a different Power Move. I find that it helps to write them out on a piece of paper. After shuffling, place the entire deck facedown on the ground, and flip over the top card. Whatever number it is, that's how many reps you do of the assigned move: If you've designated hearts as push-ups, then the 7 of hearts means you do 7 push-ups. Continue to flip through the deck card by card and perform each move to the number on the card. Just like in certain regular card games, jacks are 11, queens are 12, and kings are 13; in this case, aces are 15.

Power Moves that involve timed exercises like a hold (plank, for example), a pulse (sumo squat pulse, for example), or cardio (jumping jacks, for example) don't work so well in this format. I mean, 1 jumping jack? One second of plank? Not in my Power Game, you don't! So assign those types of exercises as the Joker card and perform thirty seconds of that move when this bonus card is flipped!

HOW TO PLAY WITH A PARTNER

This is a great game to play with a workout buddy. Take turns flipping over the cards, and feel free to place blame on whoever turns over the hardest ones!

HOW TO MODIFY FOR YOUR FITNESS LEVEL

MODIFY DOWN

- Remove the jacks, queens, kings, and aces from the deck so you only have numeral cards.
- Use the ace as a 1 rather than a 15.

MODIFY UP

- For pulse, hold, or cardio moves, add a zero to the number on the card. For example, the 2 of clubs is 20 seconds. This makes the ace of clubs 150 seconds. Wowzers!
- Both jokers are assigned exercises for 60 to 90 seconds, like mountain climbers, skater hops, plank jacks, plank frog jumps, elbow plank hip dips, flutter kicks, jumping jacks, high knees, or running in place.

Get creative with your combinations and push yourself to have as little rest as possible.

MY FAVORITE POWER MOVE COMBINATIONS

#1

♣ **CLUBS:** Floor dips

♦ **DIAMONDS:** Jumping lunges

♥ **HEARTS:** Push-ups

♠ **SPADES:** Squats

#2

♣ **CLUBS:** Reverse lunges with left leg

♦ **DIAMONDS:** Reverse lunges with right leg

♥ **HEARTS:** Biceps curls

♠ **SPADES:** Shoulder presses

#3

♣ **CLUBS:** Squats into lunge left

♦ **DIAMONDS:** Squats into lunge right

♥ **HEARTS:** Chest presses

♠ **SPADES:** Overhead triceps extensions

#4

♣ **CLUBS:** Jumping lunges

♦ **DIAMONDS:** Military push-ups

♥ **HEARTS:** Bent over rows

♠ **SPADES:** Lateral raises

#5

♣ **CLUBS:** Lateral lunges on left

♦ **DIAMONDS:** Lateral lunges on right

♥ **HEARTS:** Plank chest taps

♠ **SPADES:** Lateral raises

Power Game #4: Roll the Dice

With Hit the Deck, you know what to expect for your workout because you'll eventually flip over all fifty-two cards plus the joker. With this game, however, there's no telling what's in store. You might end up getting really tough combos or you might get a break. And, of course, if it feels easy, keep going!

HOW TO PLAY

Choose six Power Moves and assign each one a number from one to six. I find that it helps to write them out on a piece of paper for easy reference. Then grab one die. You'll roll the die twice at the beginning of every round. The first number you roll is the Power Move you perform. The second number you roll is how many reps you perform or seconds you hold it for, depending on the type of move. While the exercises you do can change each time you play, always use the two lists that follow to determine how many or for how long to do them. For a complete workout, do ten to twelve rounds.

POWER MOVES WITH REPS

⚀ : 5 reps

⚁ : 10 reps

⚂ : 15 reps

⚃ : 20 reps

⚄ : 25 reps

⚅ : 30 reps

TIMED POWER MOVES

⚀ : 10 seconds

⚁ : 20 seconds

⚂ : 30 seconds

⚃ : 40 seconds

⚄ : 50 seconds

⚅ : 60 seconds

HOW TO PLAY WITH A PARTNER

Work together to choose six moves that are challenging to both of you. And when you're ready to start playing, take turns rolling the die—one person rolls it both times the first round, the other person rolls it both times the second round, and so forth.

HOW TO MODIFY FOR YOUR FITNESS LEVEL

MODIFY DOWN
- Reduce the number of reps.
- For timed moves, cut the number of seconds in half.

MODIFY UP
Increase the total number of rounds you do. Start at 10 and see how high you can go each workout!

MY FAVORITE POWER MOVE COMBINATIONS

#1 (REPS)

1: Squats

2: Push-ups

3: Sit-ups

4: Floor dips

5: Reverse lunges with left leg

6: Reverse lunges with right leg

#2 (REPS)

1: Jumping lunges

2: Biceps curls

3: Shoulder presses

4: Bridge pulses

5: Table slides left leg

6: Table slides right leg

#3 (REPS)

1: Hammer curls

2: Lateral raises

3: Triceps kickbacks

4: Chest presses

5: Squat side kicks left

6: Squat side kicks right

#4 (TIMED)

1: Plank jacks

2: Mountain climbers

3: Sumo squats

4: Jump rope

5: Squat holds

6: Plank

#5 (TIMED)

1: Plank frog jumps

2: Hammer curls

3: W pulses

4: Skater hops

5: Fire hydrant pulses left

6: Fire hydrant pulses right

Power Game #5: TV GAMES

Every time you sit on your couch to watch TV, you're missing an easy opportunity to work out. In the spirit of drinking games—my kids tell me that this is a thing (I have NO prior knowledge whatsoever)—turn your viewing routine into a workout.

HOW TO PLAY

Create at least five rules to follow for the entire show. Use a variety of Power Moves and assign each a number of reps that is challenging to you.

HOW TO PLAY WITH A PARTNER

Create the rules together, using your knowledge of the show and your personal preferences of exercises.

HOW TO MODIFY TO YOUR FITNESS LEVEL

MODIFY DOWN
Limit this game to a half-hour show.
Start with a small number of reps, like 5 push-ups rather than 15.

MODIFY UP
Add weights to moves that don't use them or increase the amount of weight for ones that do.
Try an hours-long televised event, like an awards show or championship game.

MY FAVORITE POWER MOVE COMBINATIONS

FOR ANY SHOW

Do jumping jacks during the opening credits.

Hold a plank for one full commercial during each break (if you're feeling up for a challenge, do a plank for the ENTIRE commercial break!).

Finish the show with mountain climbers until the next show begins. Or start doing squat jumps as soon as the end credits begin all the way until they finish.

FOR A REALITY SHOW

Every time someone talks directly to the camera

Every time a contestant cries or gets emotional

Every time there's a voice-over

FOR A SITCOM

Every time you hear a laugh track

Every time there's a scene change

FOR MORNING-NEWS SHOWS

Every time there is breaking news

Every time they tell you the weather

FOR A DRAMA

Every time dramatic music plays

FOR A SPORTING EVENT

Every time either team or player scores

Every time there is a penalty

FOR AN AWARDS SHOW

Every time a winner is announced

Every time a montage is shown

Every time a host changes outfits

Every time an acceptance speech involves tears

Every time there's a standing ovation

Now that you have an idea of how Power Games work, take time to plan your workouts like you do your meals. You've heard it before—if you fail to plan, plan to fail. Instead, plan to succeed, then hold yourself accountable. Work with a trainer, work out with a friend, join a support group, or use apps like my Pretty Muscles app to help you! These are great ways to hold yourself accountable and get all the benefits these workouts have to offer.

10

POWER PLATES
FOR LIFE

You are awesome. No—you're super-awesome!

You made it through the four weeks of Power Plates. Congratulations!

In just one month, you've learned and applied a balanced, effective way of eating and exercise—one that is now resistant to weight gain because of its anti-inflammatory power. Your dedication has paid off. This is a huge, important accomplishment, something that many others have failed to achieve.

Now the important thing is that you stay true to the Power Plates lifestyle.

I have to be really honest at this point in the book. You will need—and I hope, want—to follow Power Plates for life. The Power Plate Diet is not only designed to get you in great shape, but it's also designed to keep you there and maintain your weight loss. Here's how to make that happen.

Stay Forever True to Power Plates Nutrition

Continue to eat five Power Plate–approved meals daily: breakfast, mid-morning snack, lunch, midafternoon snack, and dinner. Follow the Power Plates template and plug in recipes that have become your favorites.

Choose mostly anti-inflammatory foods like those I've listed in this book in order to keep your body fat-proofed.

Properly combine your meals. At every meal, have a lean protein, a carbohydrate, veggies, and some fat. Eating a lot of lean protein at meals may help you maintain your weight loss, because protein can help reduce appetite and promote fullness. To me, protein is an amazing, natural appetite suppressant and fat-burner.

As for carbs, limiting your carb intake in the evening may also help you maintain your weight loss. So continue to do my Modified Carb Fast as part of the plan. A friendly reminder: Starchy carbs are fine at breakfast and lunch; lower starch foods are nice at dinner, but no grains. This will keep your blood sugar from spiking then crashing, plus help your body burn fat.

Keep eating plenty of non-starchy veggies! Lots of research links high vegetable intake to better weight control. You can eat fairly hefty portions without putting on weight and take in an impressive amount of nutrients. Remember that vegetables are loaded with fiber, which makes you feel full and offers wonderful health benefits.

Stay Consistent

Consistency is a big deal when it comes to keeping your weight off or reaching your goals. One of the most important ways to be consistent is to live the four clean habits: Ease back on sugar, don't eat starchy carbs after 3 or 4 p.m., watch your alcohol intake, and minimize sodium in your diet. These are simple, sustainable changes to your lifestyle.

Plus, these healthy habits will become second nature when you get used to them. Eventually, creating Power Plates will be effortless, and you'll be able to maintain your weight easily. But you can still enjoy your favorites in moderation! This is a forever lifestyle, not a diet.

Water Your Body

Continue to take in lots of water—remember that the goal is to drink half your body weight in ounces each day.

Drinking plenty of water helps you keep weight off—for three reasons. First, it promotes fullness, especially if you drink a glass or two before meals. Second, drinking water burns fat. It slightly increases the amount of calories you expend throughout the day. In one study, drinking just two eight-ounce glasses of water bumped up metabolic rate by 30 percent! The researchers then calculated that drinking a half gallon of water daily could burn off approximately a hundred calories—about the same amount you'd burn off during a brisk fifteen-minute walk. Your metabolism will kick into gear—let's get this engine running! Third, water flushes toxins from the body that can cause inflammation and block weight loss.

Water is certainly more than a thirst quencher!

Practice "Strategic Cheating"

You're allowed to indulge yourself at one MEAL or two each week. Remember it's not a whole cheat day—you've worked too hard! You might want to do this over the weekend. Wouldn't you agree that weekends have never been kind to dieters? Life changes on the weekends. You TGIF on Fridays. You go to parties, celebrations, and other get-togethers. You might even hit a Sunday brunch. Most of us can stay pretty disciplined during the week, so why not loosen up a bit over the weekend? Just don't go overboard or look at the weekend as a free-for-all. This used to be me! Weekends were my jam for years and as a consequence I wasn't getting the results I truly wanted. It was only when I found moderation through the weekends that I stopped ruining my hard work throughout the week.

Stay Active

Several studies have found that people who do the equivalent of thirty minutes a day of exercise, after losing weight, are more likely to maintain their weight. The takeaway: Do your Tabata workouts three or four times every week, and have fun performing my Power Game workouts. You should also be walking as much as you can, with the goal of 10,000 steps daily, or about five miles. Use a fitness tracker to keep track of your progress and to motivate yourself to increase that number every day.

If you get super-busy during the week, take advantage of your extra time on the weekends. Use it to do more physical activity. Even weekend chores such as gardening, doing housework, painting, bagging grass, shoveling snow, helping your kid move to college—all burn a boatload of calories. Exercising, whether with standard workouts or lifestyle activities, is a fantastic way to maintain a lean and fit body.

Check In with Your Weight

As I've said, I'm not a big fan of stepping on scales. However, weighing yourself periodically can be helpful for weight maintenance. This is because it keeps you in check with whether you're gaining, losing, or holding the line, as well as encouraging positive weight-control habits. I think it's equally useful to observe whether your clothes are starting to feel tight. If you see a trend, not a short-term fluctuation, then reevaluate your choices following my Power Plates principles. It's a whole lot easier to lose a little than a lot.

TROUBLE-SHOOTING MAINTENANCE

If you find that pounds are creeping back on, do the following reality check:

1. Review your meals to make sure you're creating Power Plates according to my guidelines.
2. Make sure you're properly combining your foods.
3. Are you eating starchy carbs at night?
4. How much water are you drinking daily?
5. Take time to evaluate your weekly fat-burning activity. How many times a week are you performing Power Moves?
6. Review the reasons you want to stay in shape and at your ideal weight—and the benefits of doing so.
7. Are you getting your daily steps in? Hit a consistent 10,000 steps!
8. Are you overindulging on the weekends?

If you can take yourself through these steps, honestly assessing your eating patterns and behavior, your weight struggles are as good as won—forever.

Structure Your Life Going Forward

Nearly twenty years into my career as an elite personal trainer, I believe more than ever in the power of having a daily routine, especially during the week. This shouldn't totally surprise you—you'll hear many fitness experts encouraging a structured routine as a way to boost energy and productivity levels. But I'm also telling you this from the perspective of a mom, a wife, and a working professional: Making smart decisions about how you'll go about your day can be one of the healthiest things you can do for your body, for your mind, and for those around you. That's because what you accomplish in a day can determine the fate of your week, your month—and even your life.

Structure powers up your mind and sets the tone for a positive, productive day. A daily routine won't look exactly the same for every person, and it might not even look exactly the same for *you* from day to day. I wrote this book for you to use as a road map to find your own version of power living. But generally speaking, before you walk out the door for the day, it's good to know what your goals are for the next twenty-four hours.

I think of every day as a game of dominoes. The second you wake up, you knock over that first tile, which knocks over the tile next to it, and so on. The choices you make, starting in the morning and continuing through the day, set in motion a series of events, directly and indirectly affecting every other part of your day. You have the ability to knock over that first domino exactly how and when you want to; however you do it, it will affect the remaining tiles of your day.

You see, your body thrives on structure. Have you ever noticed that you tend to feel more alert, hungry, or ready for a nap around the same time every day? We are driven by our circadian rhythm, which is a twenty-four-hour hormonal cycle that tells your body what to do—wake up, eat, sleep, repeat—and when to do it. It's like a built-in alarm clock. Waking up and going to bed around the same time every day, weekends included, are crucial for keeping your circadian rhythm in check. Your circadian rhythm even affects bodily functions like digestion, as well as your levels of concentration and productivity. When it's functioning properly, your body works more efficiently and overall you feel more energized.

I didn't always love the idea of a structured day—especially growing up, when I wanted to be rebellious—but that changed when I enlisted in the military and went to basic training. In boot camp, you really have no choice but to follow orders! The subsequent nine years I spent in the Marine Corps only strengthened my appreciation of setting a routine and following it every day. It's been part of my life ever since.

I suggest that you draw a road map of how you'd like your day to look, and some days, you might even include a to-do list. When you wake up without a set plan for the morning, you're inviting unnecessary stress into your life. And stress will inflame your body!

Making important decisions on the fly can be dangerous because you often default to the easiest answer: what to eat for breakfast (leftover pizza!), what to pack for lunch (a sodium-filled frozen meal!), when to work out (oops, not enough time today!). A solid routine takes the guesswork out of these frantic moments, allowing you to move through your daily motions in a calmer, more relaxed way.

My weekdays are jam-packed from 4 a.m. to 10 p.m., and I don't slow down much on the weekends. I get asked a lot how I make it all work. There is only one way it *can* work: routines, structure, and planning ahead. I can be a bit of a bear if my routine gets messed up. Just ask my family! But that adherence to structure has allowed me to be successful, healthy, and able to grab more opportunities. I swear by it.

And while a daily structure can be great "me time"—because you're primarily doing it for your own health and sanity—it can also make for great family time. I started teaching my kids about the values of a routine when they were young. I suggest having a routine in place for yourself and, once you have mastered that, creating one for the rest of the household. Just like the Power Plates lifestyle described in this book, it's all about moderation.

I'm no strict tyrant, but I don't allow laziness in my household, either. (Trying to create this all at once can be overwhelming, so take it one step at a time!) If you live with other people—big ones or little ones—you know that chaos feeds off of chaos. As soon as one person's day gets derailed, they risk bringing everyone else down with them. Fortunately, the opposite is also true. If you feel levelheaded and prepared, you will be better able to lead your partner, kids, or roommates through whatever the day throws your way.

I prefer "habits" and "routines" over hard-and-fast "rules"—living a clean and lean lifestyle doesn't mean you can never eat pizza or that you have to do the same workout every day. A life full of rules, in my eyes, is just setting yourself up for failure because it's simply not sustainable and it's really boring. A routine, on the other hand, has room for flexibility, so while you'll get into a groove, you're not necessarily doing the exact same thing every day.

A routine will also help you master self-discipline, if that's something you've been struggling with. Eventually each task in your routine becomes easier and more familiar. Keep it positive: Don't think of a routine as "I *can't* do all *these* things"—think of it as "I *can* do *these* things one at a time."

So, if you put in the effort and commit to the Power Plates lifestyle beyond these four weeks, what will you get out of it? The benefits are both physical and mental, both short-term and long-term. With the momentum you've already created, you'll find yourself making smarter choices throughout the day, having more energy, and being more alert.

It takes around three weeks to create new habits and by this point—four weeks in—you likely won't have to think about each step because Power Plates is your new normal. Thanks to consistent anti-inflammatory nutrition and movement, you should be feeling great, physically. Your joints will feel better throughout the day, you'll feel less light-headed during workouts, and you'll experience fewer cramps when running.

You should continue to notice improvements in your overall health and energy level, including your weight loss if you're being consistent. Your muscle strength will increase, and so will your desire to move, your craving to be healthy, and your desire to stick with this lifestyle.

My Final Words of Motivation

I consider myself lucky because I've always seen health and fitness as something to celebrate. I often think of all the people who can't move whenever they want to—I can barely handle it when I'm out of commission for a day or two due to an injury! But I realize everybody is different and it might take a while to reach this point of gratefulness. If it helps, consider writing this down and making it your mantra: I don't *have* to exercise and eat healthy, I *get* to exercise and eat healthy. It's not a punishment, it's a reward.

These four weeks have just been the beginning. You'll need to continue living the four Power Plates habits, the anti-inflammatory nutrition, and the high-intensity workouts. Backsliding into old damaging habits will take you back to square one. Who wants that? Not you! Once a Power Plates follower, always a Power Plates follower.

REFERENCES

INTRODUCTION

Hammerling, U., et al. 2016. Consumption of Red/Processed Meat and Colorectal Carcinoma: Possible Mechanisms Underlying the Significant Association. *Critical Reviews in Food Science and Nutrition* 56: 614–634.

1: BE FAT-PROOF!

Deng, T., et al. 2013. Class II major histocompatibility complex plays an essential role in obesity-induced adipose inflammation. *Cell Metabolism* 17: 411–422.

Ebbling, C.B., et al. 2012. Effects of dietary composition on energy expenditure during weight-loss maintenance. *JAMA* 307: 2627–2634.

Gammone, M.A., et al. 2018. Omega-3 Polyunsaturated Fatty Acids: Benefits and Endpoints in Sport. *Nutrients* 11: E46.

Kershaw, E.E., and Flier, I.S. 2004. Adipose tissue as an endocrine organ. *Journal of Clinical Endocrinology* 89: 2548–2556.

Lonnie, M., et al. 2018. Protein for Life: Review of Optimal Protein Intake, Sustainable Dietary Sources and the Effect on Appetite in Ageing Adults. *Nutrients* 10: E360.

Martens, M.J., et al. 2011. A solid high-protein meal evokes stronger hunger suppression than a liquefied high-protein meal. *Obesity* 19: 522–527.

Murakami, S. 2015. Role of taurine in the pathogenesis of obesity. *Molecular Nutrition & Food Research* 59: 1353–1363.

Nicole, M., et al. 2008. Evidence for sugar addiction: Behavioral and neurochemical effects of intermittent, excessive sugar intake. *Neuroscience and Biobehavioral Reviews* 32: 20–39.

Parolini, C. 2019. Effects of Fish n-3 PUFAs on Intestinal Microbiota and Immune System. *Marine Drugs* 17: E374.

Raatz, S. The Question of Sugar, www.ars.usda.gov, accessed February 2020.

Rebello. C.J., et al. 2013. Dietary strategies to increase satiety. *Advances in Food and Nutrition Research* 69: 105–182.

Rosa, F.T., et al. 2014. Oxidative stress and inflammation in obesity after taurine supplementation: a double-blind, placebo-controlled study. *European Journal of Nutrition* 53: 823–830.

Slaving, J.L., 2005. Dietary fiber and body weight. *Nutrition* 21: 411–418.

Spalding, K.L., et al. 2008. Dynamics of fat cell turnover in humans. *Nature* 453: 783–787.

Stenkula, K.G., and Erlanson-Albertson, C. 2018. Adipose cell size: importance in health and disease. *American Journal of Physiology, Regulatory, Integrative, and Comparative Physiology* 315: R284–R295.

Suter, P.M. 2005. Carbohydrates and dietary fiber. *Handbook of Experimental Pharmacology* 170: 231–261.

Tchernof, A., and Despres, J.P. 2013 Pathophysiology of human visceral obesity: an update. *Physiological Reviews* 93: 359–404.

Zhu, F., et al. 2018. Anti-inflammatory effects of phytochemicals from fruits, vegetables, and food legumes: A review. *Critical Reviews in Food Science and Nutrition* 58: 1260–1270.

2: THE WEIGHT-INFLAMMATION CONNECTION

American Cancer Society. 2020. Cancer statistics, cancer.org.

Basta, G., et al. 2004. Advanced glycation end products and vascular inflammation: implications for accelerated atherosclerosis in diabetes. *Cardiovascular Research* 63: 582–592.

Bruun, J.M., et al. 2015. Consumption of sucrose-sweetened soft drinks increases plasma levels of uric acid in overweight and obese subjects: a 6-month randomised controlled trial. *European Journal of Clinical Nutrition* 69: 949–953.

DiNicolantonio, J.J., et al. 2018. Fructose-induced inflammation and increased cortisol: A new mechanism for how sugar induces visceral adiposity. *Progress in Cardiovascular Disease* 61: 3–9.

Engin, A. 2017. Adiponectin-Resistance in Obesity. *Advances in Experimental Medicine and Biology* 960: 415–441.

Furman, D., et al. 2019. Chronic inflammation in the etiology of disease across the life span. *Nature Medicine* 25: 1822–1832.

Glushakova, O., et al. 2008. Fructose induces the inflammatory molecule ICAM-1 in endothelial cells. *Journal of the American Society of Nephrology* 19: 1712–1720.

Hammerling, U., et al. 2016. Consumption of Red/Processed Meat and Colorectal

Carcinoma: Possible Mechanisms Underlying the Significant Association. *Critical Reviews in Food Science and Nutrition* 56: 614–634.

Larsson, S.C., et al. 2006. Processed meat consumption, dietary nitrosamines and stomach cancer risk in a cohort of Swedish women. *International Journal of Cancer* 119: 915–919.

Pahwa. R., et al. 2019. *Chronic Inflammation* by R. Pahwa, et al. published by StatPearls.

Phillips, C.M., et al. 2019. Dietary Inflammatory Index and Non-Communicable Disease Risk: A Narrative Review. *Nutrients* 11: E1873.

Raphaelle, L., et al. 2008. Processed meat and colorectal cancer: a review of epidemiologic and experimental evidence. *Nutrition and Cancer* 60: 131–144.

Renata, M., et al. 2010. Red and processed meat consumption and risk of incident coronary heart disease, stroke, and diabetes: A systematic review and meta-analysis. *Circulation* 121: 2271–2283.

Seth, D., et al. 2020. Food Allergy: A Review. *Pediatric Annals* 49: e50–e58.

Suez, J., et al. 2014. Artificial sweeteners induce glucose intolerance by altering the gut microbiota. *Nature* 514: 181–186.

Tuck, C.J., et al. 2019. Food Intolerances. *Nutrients* 11: E1684.

Uribarri, J., et al. 2010. Advanced glycation end products in foods and a practical guide to their reduction in the diet. *Journal of the American Dietetic Association* 110: 911–916.

3: CLEAN EATING

Garaulet, M., et al. 2013. Timing of food intake predicts weight loss effectiveness. *International Journal of Obesity* 37: 604–611.

Jakubowicz, D., et al. 2013. High caloric intake at breakfast vs. dinner differentially influences weight loss of overweight and obese women. *Obesity* 21: 2504–2512.

Jung, S.M., et al. 2019. Sodium Chloride Aggravates Arthritis via Th17 Polarization. *Yonsei Medical Journal* 60: 88–97.

4: TORCH FAT WITH POWER FOODS

Blesso, C.N., and Fernandez, M.L. 2018. Dietary Cholesterol, Serum Lipids, and Heart Disease: Are Eggs Working for or Against You? *Nutrients* 10: E426.

Kahleova, H., et al. 2018. A plant-based diet in overweight individuals in a 16-week randomized clinical trial: metabolic benefits of plant protein. *Nutrition & Diabetes* 8: 58.

Kleiner, S.M. 1999. Water: an essential but overlooked nutrient. *Journal of the American Dietetic Association* 99: 200–206.

Lucas, L., et al. 2011. Molecular mechanisms of inflammation. Anti-inflammatory benefits of virgin olive oil and the phenolic compound oleocanthal. *Current Pharmaceutical Design* 17: 754–768.

Ramel, A., et al. 2009. Consumption of cod and weight loss in young overweight and obese adults on an energy reduced diet for 8 weeks. *Nutrition, Metabolism & Cardiovascular Diseases* 19: 690–696.

Ramel, A., et al. 2010. Effects of weight loss and seafood consumption on inflammation parameters in young, overweight and obese European men and women during 8 weeks of energy restriction. *European Journal of Clinical Nutrition* 64: 987–993.

Simental-Mendía, M., et al. 2019. Efficacy and safety of avocado-soybean unsaponifiables for the treatment of hip and knee osteoarthritis: A systematic review and meta-analysis of randomized placebo-controlled trials. *International Journal of Rheumatic Diseases* 22: 1607–1615.

Tan, S.Y., et al. 2014. A review of the effects of nuts on appetite, food intake, metabolism, and body weight. *American Journal of Clinical Nutrition* 100 Supplement 1: 412S–422S.

Tapesell, L.C., et al. 2006. Health benefits of herbs and spices: the past, the present, the future. *The Medical Journal of Australia* 185: S1–S24.

Thorsdottir, N., et al. 2007. Randomized trial of weight-loss-diets for young adults varying in fish and fish oil content. *International Journal of Obesity* 31: 1560–1566.

Turner-McGrievy, G., et al. 2017. A plant-based diet for overweight and obesity prevention and treatment. *Journal of Geriatric Cardiology* 14: 369–374.

Vander Wal, J.S., et al. 2008. Egg breakfast enhances weight loss. *International Journal of Obesity* 32: 1545–1551.

Vander Wal, J.S., et al. 2005. Short-term effect of eggs on satiety in overweight and obese subjects. *Journal of the American College of Nutrition* 24: 510–515.

Xu, Y., et al. 2018. Whole grain diet reduces systemic inflammation: A meta-analysis of 9 randomized trials. *Medicine* 97: e12995.

5: CREATE POUND-DROPPING MEALS

Figueres Juher, T., and Basés Pérez, E. 2015. An overview of the beneficial effects of hydrolysed collagen intake on joint and bone health and on skin ageing. *Nutrición Hospitalaria* 32 Supplement 1: 62–66.

Hetherington, M.M., et al. 2018. Understanding the science of portion control and the art of downsizing. *The Proceedings of the Nutrition Society* 77: 347–355.

Hexsel, D., et al. 2017. Oral supplementation with specific bioactive collagen peptides improves nail growth and reduces symptoms of brittle nails. *Journal of Cosmetic Dermatology* 16: 520–526.

Kodentsova, V.M., et al. 2015. Vitamin-mineral supplements in nutrition of adults. *Voprosy Pitaniia* 84: 141–150.

McCormick, D.B. 2010. Vitamin/mineral supplements: of questionable benefit for the general population. *Nutrition Reviews* 68: 207–213.

Proksch, E., et al. 2014. Oral supplementation of specific collagen peptides has beneficial effects on human skin physiology: a double-blind, placebo-controlled study. *Skin Pharmacology and Physiology* 27: 47–55.

8: POWER MOVES

Editor. Risks of physical inactivity, www.hopkinsmedicine.org/healthlibrary/conditions/cardiovascular_diseases/risks_of_physical_inactivity_85,p00218.

9: POWER GAMES

Tabata, I. 2019. Tabata training: one of the most energetically effective high-intensity intermittent training methods. *The Journal of Physiological Sciences* 69: 559–572.

Tabata, I., et al. 1996. Effects of moderate-intensity endurance and high-intensity intermittent training on anaerobic capacity and VO$_2$max. *Medicine and Science in Sports and Exercise* 28: 1327–1330.

10: POWER PLATES FOR LIFE

Boschmann, M., et al. 2003. Water-induced thermogenesis. *Journal of Clinical Endocrinology and Metabolism* 88: 6015–6019.

Dennis, E.A., et al. 2010. Water consumption increases weight loss during a hypocaloric diet intervention in middle-aged and older adults. *Obesity* 18: 300–307.

Dominik, H.P, and Varman, T.S. 2104. A high-protein diet for reducing body fat: mechanisms and possible caveats. *Nutrition & Metabolism* 11: 53.

Halton, T.L., and Hu, F.B. 2004. The effects of high protein diets on thermogenesis, satiety and weight loss: a critical review. *Journal of the American College of Nutrition* 23: 373–385.

Rosenbaum, M., and Leibel, R.L. 2010. Adaptive thermogenesis in humans. *International Journal of Obesity* 34: S47–S55.

Soeliman, F.A., and Azadbakht, L. 2104. Weight loss maintenance: A review on dietary related strategies. *Journal of Research in Medical Sciences* 19: 268–275.

Swift, D.L., et al. 2014. The role of exercise and physical activity in weight loss and maintenance. *Progress in Cardiovascular Diseases* 56: 441–447.

Tapsell, L.C., et al. 2014. Weight loss effects from vegetable intake: a 12-month randomised controlled trial. *European Journal of Clinical Nutrition* 68: 778–785.

Westerterp-Plantenga, M.S., et al. 2009. Dietary protein, weight loss, and weight maintenance. *Annual Review of Nutrition* 29: 21–41.

Wing, R.R., and Phelan, S. 2005. Long-term weight loss maintenance. *American Journal of Clinical Nutrition* 82 (1 Supplement): 222S–225S.

ACKNOWLEDGMENTS

Neil Whitney—who has been an amazing sounding board.

Ann Stewart—my mom, who has always been a solid rock in my life.

My amazing clients—who hear all and provide some of the greatest feedback!

Sean—my biggest cheerleader and best friend. He's lucky to have married me.

Hunter and Hayden—my kids, who have been patient through good times and stressful times.

Thank you to all those in my life who challenged, lifted, educated, and supported me through the making of this book and beyond!

INDEX

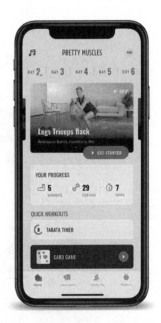
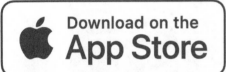
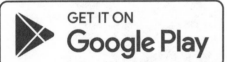
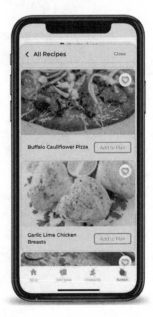

Also by

ERIN OPREA

"Erin's approach is simple and realistic. The more you apply her principles of food and exercise, the more success you will have." —**JENNIFER NETTLES**

THE

4×4

DIET

4 **KEY FOODS**   4 **MINUTE WORKOUTS**

— FOUR WEEKS TO —
THE BODY YOU WANT

ERIN OPREA

HARMONY
BOOKS • NEW YORK

Available wherever books are sold